Review and Assessment of the Health and Productivity Benefits of Green Schools: An Interim Report

Committee to Review and Assess the Health and Productivity Benefits of Green Schools
Board on Infrastructure and the Constructed Environment
Division on Engineering and Physical Sciences

NATIONAL RESEARCH COUNCIL
OF THE NATIONAL ACADEMIES

THE NATIONAL ACADEMIES PRESS
WASHINGTON, D.C.
www.nap.edu

THE NATIONAL ACADEMIES PRESS 500 Fifth Street, N.W. Washington, DC 20001

NOTICE: The project that is the subject of this report was approved by the Governing Board of the National Research Council, whose members are drawn from the councils of the National Academy of Sciences, the National Academy of Engineering, and the Institute of Medicine. The members of the committee responsible for the report were chosen for their special competences and with regard for appropriate balance.

This study was supported by a Master Services Agreement between the National Academy of Sciences and the Massachusetts Technology Collaborative (awarded November 2004); Grant 1906 between the Barr Foundation and the National Academy of Sciences (awarded September 2004); and funding from the Connecticut Clean Energy Fund (awarded April 2005); the Kendall Foundation (awarded March 2005); and the U.S. Green Building Council (awarded February 2005). Any opinions, findings, conclusions, or recommendations expressed in this publication are those of the author(s) and do not necessarily reflect the views of the organizations or agencies that provided support for the project.

International Standard Book Number 0-309-10120-4

Copies of this report are available from the Board on Infrastructure and the Constructed Environment, National Research Council, 500 Fifth Street, N.W., Room 943, Washington, DC 20001; (202) 334-3376.

Additional copies of this report are available from the National Academies Press, 500 Fifth Street, N.W., Lockbox 285, Washington, DC 20055; (800) 624-6242 or (202) 334-3313 (in the Washington metropolitan area); Internet, http://www.nap.edu.

Printed in the United States of America

THE NATIONAL ACADEMIES

Advisers to the Nation on Science, Engineering, and Medicine

The **National Academy of Sciences** is a private, nonprofit, self-perpetuating society of distinguished scholars engaged in scientific and engineering research, dedicated to the furtherance of science and technology and to their use for the general welfare. Upon the authority of the charter granted to it by the Congress in 1863, the Academy has a mandate that requires it to advise the federal government on scientific and technical matters. Dr. Ralph J. Cicerone is president of the National Academy of Sciences.

The **National Academy of Engineering** was established in 1964, under the charter of the National Academy of Sciences, as a parallel organization of outstanding engineers. It is autonomous in its administration and in the selection of its members, sharing with the National Academy of Sciences the responsibility for advising the federal government. The National Academy of Engineering also sponsors engineering programs aimed at meeting national needs, encourages education and research, and recognizes the superior achievements of engineers. Dr. Wm. A. Wulf is president of the National Academy of Engineering.

The **Institute of Medicine** was established in 1970 by the National Academy of Sciences to secure the services of eminent members of appropriate professions in the examination of policy matters pertaining to the health of the public. The Institute acts under the responsibility given to the National Academy of Sciences by its congressional charter to be an adviser to the federal government and, upon its own initiative, to identify issues of medical care, research, and education. Dr. Harvey V. Fineberg is president of the Institute of Medicine.

The **National Research Council** was organized by the National Academy of Sciences in 1916 to associate the broad community of science and technology with the Academy's purposes of furthering knowledge and advising the federal government. Functioning in accordance with general policies determined by the Academy, the Council has become the principal operating agency of both the National Academy of Sciences and the National Academy of Engineering in providing services to the government, the public, and the scientific and engineering communities. The Council is administered jointly by both Academies and the Institute of Medicine. Dr. Ralph J. Cicerone and Dr. Wm. A. Wulf are chair and vice chair, respectively, of the National Research Council.

www.national-academies.org

COMMITTEE TO REVIEW AND ASSESS THE HEALTH AND PRODUCTIVITY BENEFITS OF GREEN SCHOOLS

JOHN D. SPENGLER, Harvard University, *Chair*
VIVIAN E. LOFTNESS, Carnegie Mellon University, *Vice Chair*
CHARLENE W. BAYER, Georgia Institute of Technology
JOHN S. BRADLEY, National Research Council, Ottawa, Canada
GLEN I. EARTHMAN, Virginia Polytechnic Institute and State University
PEYTON A. EGGLESTON, Johns Hopkins University
PAUL FISETTE, University of Massachusetts, Amherst
CAROLINE BREESE HALL, University of Rochester
GARY T. HENRY, Georgia State University
CLIFFORD S. MITCHELL, Johns Hopkins University
MARK S. REA, Rensselaer Polytechnic Institute
HENRY SANOFF, North Carolina State University
CAROL H. WEISS, Harvard University
SUZANNE M. WILSON, Michigan State University

Staff

LYNDA STANLEY, Director, Board on Infrastructure and the Constructed Environment
KEVIN LEWIS, Program Officer
PAT WILLIAMS, Senior Project Assistant

Acknowledgment of Reviewers

This interim report has been reviewed in draft form by individuals chosen for their diverse perspectives and technical expertise, in accordance with procedures approved by the NRC's Report Review Committee. The purpose of this independent review is to provide candid and critical comments that will assist the institution in making its published report as sound as possible and to ensure that the report meets institutional standards for objectivity, evidence, and responsiveness to the study charge. The review comments and draft manuscript remain confidential to protect the integrity of the deliberative process. We wish to thank the following individuals for their review of this report:

Karen Anderson, Florida Department of Health,
William J. Fisk, Lawrence Berkeley National Laboratory,
Robert E. Fullilove, Columbia University,
Martin Moeck, Pennsylvania State University, and
William Rose, University of Illinois at Urbana-Champaign.

Although the reviewers listed above have provided many constructive comments and suggestions, they were not asked to endorse the conclusions or recommendations, nor did they see the final draft of the report before its release. The review of this report was overseen by Henry W. Riecken, University of Pennsylvania, Emeritus, and Richard N. Wright, National Institute of Standards and Technology, retired. Appointed by the National Research Council, they were responsible for making certain that an independent examination of this report was carried out in accordance with institutional procedures and that all review comments were carefully considered. Responsibility for the final content of this report rests entirely with the authoring committee and the institution.

Contents

EXECUTIVE SUMMARY 1

1 INTRODUCTION 8
Green Schools Versus Conventional New Schools, 9
The Element of Time, 9
Modeling the Effects of Green Schools, 10
Complexity of the Task, 13
Committee's Approach, 16
Findings, 19

2 BUILDING ENVELOPE, MOISTURE MANAGEMENT, AND HEALTH 20
Building Envelope and Moisture Management, 20
Excessive Moisture and Health, 21
Findings and Recommendation, 24

3 VENTILATION, POLLUTANT SOURCE CONTROL, HEALTH, AND PERFORMANCE 26
Indoor Air Quality and Pollutant Source Control, 27
Indoor Air Quality and Ventilation Rates, 28
Ventilation and Health, 30
Ventilation and Comfort, 31
Moisture Management in Heating, Ventilation, and Air-Conditioning Systems, 31
Findings, 32

4 LIGHTING, PERFORMANCE, AND HEALTH 34
Lighting and Its Impact on the Visual and Circadian Systems, 35
Daylighting and Student Learning, 37
Lighting and the Circadian System, 39
Daylighting, View, Performance, and Health, 40
Findings and Recommendations, 40

5 NOISE, ACOUSTICS, STUDENT LEARNING, AND TEACHER HEALTH 42
Noise and Student Achievement, 43
Noise and Teachers' Health, 45
Findings and Recommendation, 45

6 BUILDING CONDITION AND STUDENT ACHIEVEMENT 46
School Building Condition and Student Achievement, 47
School Building Functionality and Student Achievement, 50
Limitations of the Current Studies, 51
Finding and Recommendation, 51

REFERENCES 53

APPENDIX: BIOGRAPHIES OF COMMITTEE MEMBERS 64

ROLE OF THE BOARD ON INFRASTRUCTURE AND THE CONSTRUCTED ENVIRONMENT 69

Executive Summary

BACKGROUND

At the request of the Massachusetts Technology Collaborative (MASSTECH), the Barr and Kendall Foundations, the Connecticut Clean Energy Fund, and the U.S. Green Building Council, the National Research Council (NRC), through the Board on Infrastructure and the Constructed Environment (BICE), appointed the Committee to Review and Assess the Health and Productivity Benefits of Green Schools. The committee's charge was to "review, assess, and synthesize the results of available studies on green schools and determine the theoretical and methodological basis for the effects of green schools on student learning and teacher productivity." In the course of the study, the committee was asked to do the following:

1. Review and assess existing empirical and theoretical studies regarding the possible connections between the characteristics of "green schools" and the health and productivity of students and teachers.
2. Develop an evaluation framework for assessing the relevance and validity of individual reports that considers the possible influence of such factors as error, bias, confounding, or chance on the reported results and that integrates the overall evidence within and between diverse types of studies.
3. Report the results of this effort in a manner that will facilitate the identification of causal relationships and the subsequent implementation of beneficial practices.
4. Identify avenues of research that represent potentially valuable opportunities to leverage existing knowledge into a better understanding of the relationships between green building technologies in schools and the performance of students and teachers.

The committee, appointed in January 2005, has held four meetings. A fifth meeting will be held in January 2006, and the committee will complete its final report by April 30, 2006. This interim report has been prepared at the request of MASSTECH. MASSTECH is preparing a legislative proposal for green school guidelines, to be submitted to the Massachusetts School Building Authority in December 2005. MASSTECH has requested a summary of the committee's findings and recommendations to date as guidance in finalizing its proposal.

Because this is an interim report, it is important to note that the committee has not yet fully addressed the statement of task. The committee has developed an evaluation framework (task 2) and has reviewed and assessed *some* of the empirical and theoretical studies that address some characteristics of green schools and their associations with the health and development of students and teachers (task 1). In this interim report, the committee has dealt with five characteristics of green schools—building envelope, ventilation, lighting, acoustics, and condition—and evaluated the scientific evidence for relationships/associations with various outcomes of health, learning, and productivity (task 3). The committee plans to review and assess additional characteristics of green schools and the evidence for associations with health and development and report the results of those assessments in its final report.

To fulfill the statement of task, the committee will also synthesize the results of all of the assessments (overall task) and identify avenues of research that represent opportunities to leverage existing knowledge into a better understanding of the relationships between green building technologies in schools and the performance of students and teachers (task 4).

COMPLEXITY OF THE TASK

The charge to this committee is to review and assess existing empirical and theoretical studies on the possible connections between characteristics of green schools and the health and performance of students and teachers. Such an evaluation would ideally be based on a generally accepted definition of green schools that would convey specific architectural features, systems, and operational practices. However, there is no single, accepted definition among educational professionals, architects, and others, of what constitutes a "green school." Instead, there are many definitions with varying levels of detail for green schools (sometimes referred to as "high-performance green schools" or "high-performance schools"). The definitions typically focus on environmental or other objectives to be achieved through "green" or sustainable design processes, features, and practices. Various sets of guidelines have been developed to suggest a multitude of ways in which the objectives can be achieved to some degree. Typically the guidelines move well beyond design and engineering criteria for school buildings to address land use, processes for construction and equipment installation, and operation and maintenance practices.

The committee's task is further complicated by the fact that green schools are not standardized in their design and there are relatively few schools considered as exemplifying green design. Adding to the complexity is the need to draw on literature from a wide array of professional disciplines, including medicine, education, architecture, and engineering. These disciplines have developed differing research methodologies and criteria for determining causality. The committee also recognizes that many factors in a school as well as in a community and individual households influence the educational achievement of individuals and schools systems. Those factors or variables can be difficult to control for or measure in evidence-based studies, which, in turn, limits the inferences that can be drawn. In addition, the effects of the built environment will necessarily appear to be small, given the number of variables.

COMMITTEE'S APPROACH

Given these complexities, the committee's approach was to identify those characteristics of green schools that are typically emphasized in the current definitions and guidelines and that differ from conventional new school construction norms. The committee also identified those characteristics that potentially have a level of importance for health and learning outcomes. In this interim report, the committee focuses on the following characteristics of green school buildings and their relationships to occupant health and productivity outcomes:

- Building envelope, moisture management, and health;
- Ventilation, pollutant source control, health, and productivity;
- Lighting, performance, and health;
- Acoustics, student learning, and teacher health; and
- Building condition and student achievement.

In evaluating the scientific literature related to these topics, the committee has relied on a hierarchy of evidence for scientific inference developed by the National Academies (Box ES.1) for use in health-related studies (IOM, 1991, 1993, 1994, 1996, 1999, 2003). This hierarchy has played an important role in the committee's deliberations.

Box ES.1 National Academies' Hierarchy of Evidence for Scientific Inference in Health-Related Studies

Sufficient Evidence of a Causal Relationship: Evidence is sufficient to conclude that a causal relationship exists between the agent and the outcome. That is, the evidence fulfills the criteria for sufficient proof of an association, and in addition, satisfies evaluation criteria such as strength of association, biologic gradient, consistency of association, biologic plausibility and coherence, and temporally correct association. The finding of sufficient evidence of a causal relationship between an exposure and a health outcome does not mean that the exposure would inevitably lead to that outcome. Rather it means that the exposure can cause the outcome, at least in some people under some circumstances.

Sufficient Evidence of an Association: Evidence is sufficient to conclude that there is an association. That is, an association between the agent and the outcome has been observed in studies in which chance, bias, and confounding can be ruled out with reasonable confidence.

Limited or Suggestive Evidence of an Association: Evidence is suggestive of an association between the agent and the outcome but is limited because chance, bias, and confounding could not be ruled out with confidence. For example, at least one high-quality study shows a positive association, but the results of other studies are inconsistent.

Inadequate or Insufficient Evidence to Determine Whether or Not an Association Exists: The available studies are of insufficient quality, consistency, or statistical power to permit a conclusion about the presence or absence of an association. Alternatively, no studies exist that examine the relationship.

Limited or Suggestive Evidence of No Association: Several adequate studies are consistent in not showing an association between the agent and the outcome. A conclusion of "no association" is inevitably limited to the conditions, magnitude of exposure, and length of observation covered by the available studies.

SOURCE: IOM, 2004.

FINDINGS AND RECOMMENDATIONS

Finding 1: In its review thus far, the committee has found the following:

- There are no well-designed, evidence-based studies concerning the overall effects of green schools on the health or development of students and teachers, in part because the concept of green schools is quite new. There are, however, a few well-designed studies that examine specific building features often emphasized in green school design and the effects of these components on health and learning.
- Given the level of interaction between people and their environments and other confounding factors, establishing cause-and-effect relationships between an attribute of a school building and its effect on students, teachers, and staff is difficult. The effects of the built environment will necessarily appear to be small, given the number of variables.
- Empirical measures do not, however, necessarily capture all relevant considerations that should be applied when evaluating research results. Qualitative aspects of the environment are also important. Thus, in the committee's collective judgment, there is value in attempting to identify design features and building processes and practices that may lead to improvements in learning, health, and productivity for students, teachers, and other school staff, even if empirical results are less than robust.

Finding 2: In regard to issues related to building envelope, moisture management, and health, the committee has found the following:

- There is sufficient evidence to establish an association between moisture problems in buildings (floods, visible dampness, leaks, mold growth in spaces or in heating, ventilation, and air-conditioning [HVAC] systems) and adverse health outcomes, particularly asthma and respiratory symptoms, among children and adults.
- Excessive moisture in a building can lead to structural damage, deterioration of the performance of building systems and components, and cosmetic damage, all of which can result in increased maintenance and repair costs.
- Guidelines for green schools typically do not adequately address the design detailing, construction, and long-term maintenance of building envelopes to ensure that allergen sources are controlled, moisture is controlled, and a building is kept dry over the long term.
- Well-designed, constructed, and maintained building envelopes are critical to the control and prevention of the excessive moisture and molds that have been associated with adverse health effects in children and adults. Designing for effective moisture management will likely have benefits for the building, including lower life-cycle costs. Excellent resources for proper moisture control design include *The Moisture Control Handbook, Principles and Practices for Residential and Small Commercial Buildings* by Joseph Lstiburek and John

Carmody (1994) and *The Building Foundation Design Handbook* (ORNL, 1988), published by Oak Ridge National Laboratory.

Recommendation 1: The control of excessive moisture, dampness, and molds to protect the health of children and adults in schools and to protect the structural integrity of a building should be a key objective for green schools. MASSTECH should develop guidelines that specifically address moisture control as it relates to the design, construction, operation, and maintenance of a school building's envelope (foundations, walls, windows, and roofs); ventilation systems; and related items such as siting, landscaping, and plumbing systems.

Finding 3: In regard to ventilation, pollutant source control, health, and performance, the committee has found the following:

- Numerous pollution sources and building system characteristics affect air quality in a school. The most important determinants of indoor air quality are (1) design and operation of the ventilation system to limit the buildup of pollutants and humidity and achieve thermal comfort, (2) control of indoor sources of pollutants, and (3) control of outdoor sources of pollutants.
- There is a robust body of evidence indicating that the health of children and adults can be affected by air quality in a school.
- A growing body of evidence suggests that teacher productivity and student learning, as measured by absenteeism, may be affected by indoor air quality as well.
- Indoor pollutants and allergens from house dust mites, pet dander, cockroaches, and rodents also contribute to increased respiratory and asthma symptoms among children and adults.
- The reduction of pollutant loads, both sensory and not, has been shown to reduce the occurrence of building-associated symptoms and to improve the health and comfort of people occupying the buildings.
- Although compliance with the American Society for Heating, Refrigeration, and Air-Conditioning Engineers (ASHRAE) standards for ventilation rates may be the minimal acceptable standard for green schools, there is good evidence that increasing the ventilation rate beyond the ASHRAE standard will further improve comfort and productivity. However, an upper limit on the ventilation rates, indicating when the benefits of outside air begin to decline, has not been established.

The committee will address additional issues related to heating, ventilation, air-conditioning, and their associations with health and productivity outcomes in its final report. Until this review is completed and the results are synthesized, the committee will defer making specific recommendations.

Finding 4: In regard to lighting, performance, and health, the committee has found the following:

- Daylight is a special light source because it may provide a view (through a window), high light levels, and good color rendering, and it is ever-changing. Direct and reflected sunlight can create significant visual problems if windows, skylights, and clerestories allow in too much or too little light. However, such problems can be controlled with manual blinds and other types of window treatments.
- There is good evidence from studies of adult populations that the visual conditions in schools resulting from both electric lighting and daylighting are adequate for most children and adults.
- There is, however, concern that a significant percentage of students in classrooms do not have properly corrected eyesight, and thus, the general lighting conditions suitable for visual functioning by the average student may be inadequate for those students without properly corrected eyesight. It could be hypothesized that daylight may benefit these children by providing higher light levels and better geometries than would otherwise be present from electric lighting alone. However, the potential advantages of daylight in classrooms for improving visual performance of children with or without properly corrected eyesight has not been systematically studied.
- Because of inconsistent results and the small number of well-designed studies, there is insufficient evidence at this time to determine whether or not an association exists between daylighting and student performance.
- A growing body of evidence suggests that lighting may play an important nonvisual role in human health and well-being through the circadian system. However, the effect of light on health through circadian regulation of sleep, depression, and cell cycle has not been directly studied in children.

Recommendation 2: To determine the potential and actual performance of a lighting system, the entire system should be assessed because total performance cannot be effectively evaluated based solely on the source of illumination or on the individual components needed to create the entire lighting system.

Recommendation 3: For green schools in which the lighting strategy is to use daylight extensively, control systems that can be easily operated, such as manual blinds or other types of window treatments, should be specified in order to control excessive sunlight or glare.

Finding 5: In regard to noise, acoustics, student learning, and teacher health, the committee has found the following:

- Sufficient evidence exists to conclude that there is an association between decreased noise levels in schools and improvement in student achievement.
- Although there is strong evidence that reduced noise levels are most important for younger children because they are still developing speech discrimination, additional research is required to more precisely define possible needs for control of reverberant sound for younger children.

- Some available evidence indicates that teacher health, in regard to voice impairment, may be adversely affected by noisier environments, although the magnitude of the effect cannot currently be estimated as a function of exposure to noise.

Recommendation 4: To facilitate student learning, guidelines for green schools should include requirements to meet American National Standards Institute (ANSI) Standard S12.60, "Acoustical Performance Criteria, Design Requirements, and Guidelines for Schools."

Finding 6: In regard to building condition and student achievement, the committee has found the following:

- The body of available research is suggestive of an association between the condition of a school building and student achievement. All of the studies analyzed by the committee found that student test scores improved as the physical condition of school buildings improved. The degree of improvement of students' test scores varied across the studies, but in all cases students in buildings in better condition scored higher than students in buildings in poor condition.

Recommendation 5: Guidelines for green schools should place significant emphasis on operations and maintenance practices if potential health and productivity benefits are to be achieved and maintained over the lifetime of a building.

1

Introduction

The charge to the Committee to Review and Assess the Health and Productivity Benefits of Green Schools is to review and assess existing empirical and theoretical studies concerning the possible connections between characteristics of "green schools" and the health and performance of students and teachers. Ideally, such an evaluation would be based on a generally accepted definition of green schools that would convey specific architectural features, systems, and operational practices. However, among educational professionals, architects, engineers, and others, there is no single, accepted definition of a green school (sometimes referred to as "high-performance green schools" or "high-performance schools"). Instead, there are many definitions with varying levels of detail. The definitions typically focus on environmental or other objectives to be achieved by building in a "green" or sustainable manner. MASSTECH, for example, defines a green school as having the following three distinct attributes:

- Less costly to operate than a conventional school,
- Designed to enhance the learning and working environment, and
- Conserves important resources such as energy and water.

The Collaborative High Performance Schools Web site notes that green schools are defined by the following 13 attributes: healthy, comfortable, energy efficient, material efficient, water efficient, easy to maintain and operate, commissioned, environmentally responsive site, a building that teaches, safe and secure, community resource, stimulating architecture, and adaptable to changing needs (CHPS, 2005). Other definitions abound.

The definitions often are put into operation through various sets of guidelines for constructing green schools. The guidelines typically identify a number of ways in which the objectives can be achieved to some degree. Such guidelines have been issued by California (CHPS, 2004) and Washington state (WSBE, 2005) and are in developmental stages in Massachusetts. These guidelines move well beyond design and engineering criteria for school buildings to address land use, processes for construction and equipment installation, and operation and maintenance practices. Guidelines may include design and engineering goals such as locating schools near public transportation to reduce pollution and land development impacts; placing a building on a site to minimize its environmental impact and optimize daylighting and solar gain; designing irrigation systems and indoor plumbing systems to conserve water; designing energy and lighting systems to conserve fossil fuels and maximize the use of renewable resources; selecting materials that are nontoxic, biodegradable, and easily recycled, and that minimize the impacts on landfills and otherwise reduce waste; and creating an indoor environment that provides occupants with thermal comfort and acoustic, visual, and air quality.

Guidelines for green schools also include construction goals such as the appropriate storage of materials on construction sites to avoid water damage, the reduction of waste materials and appropriate disposal to reduce resource depletion, and the introduction of commissioning practices[1] to ensure the performance of integrated building systems. To address the life-cycle performance of schools, guidelines for operation and maintenance practices are also included, such as using nontoxic cleaning products, replacing air filters in ventilation systems on a regular schedule, and establishing a long-term indoor environmental management plan.

GREEN SCHOOLS VERSUS CONVENTIONAL NEW SCHOOLS

Given the lack of a generally accepted definition of green schools, the committee focused on differentiating land use, building design/engineering, construction, and operations and maintenance practices that are often highlighted in the green school literature and not likely to be introduced in conventional new school construction. The committee then identified research in the literature looking at the relationships between these characteristics and a performance outcome (health, learning, productivity) in students or teachers. A complicating factor is that building systems and characteristics operate in an integrated fashion to effectively deliver (or not) overall building performance in regard to thermal comfort; air, visual, acoustic, and spatial quality; and long-term building integrity. Further, this performance will be affected by the operation and maintenance of these integrated systems over time and by the occupants of buildings and their activities. Thus there is a need to synthesize the results so that potential trade-offs between certain features and practices can be identified.

The committee's approach then was to identify those building characteristics that are emphasized in available definitions and guidelines as constituting green school design and differ from conventional new school construction norms. The committee also identified those elements that potentially have a level of importance for health and learning outcomes. In this interim report, the committee has focused on the following characteristics of green school buildings and their relationship to occupant health and productivity outcomes:

- Building envelope, moisture management, and health;
- Ventilation, pollutant source control, health, and productivity;
- Lighting, performance, and health;
- Acoustics, student learning, and teacher health; and
- Building condition and student achievement.

THE ELEMENT OF TIME

The design and construction of a new school or the renovation of an existing one require a substantial commitment of resources—time, dollars, materials, expertise—by a community. Typically, once built, a school is used for educational purposes for 30 years or

[1] Commissioning is "a quality-focused process for enhancing the delivery of a project. The process focuses on verifying and documenting that the facility and all of its systems and assemblies are planned, designed, installed, tested, operated to meet the Owner's Project Requirements" (ANSI, 2004).

longer. While the building is in service, the investment made in its operation, maintenance, and repair will be six to eight times greater than the initial cost of construction.[2]

School buildings are composed of materials and components that wear out at differing rates and that vary in their complexity and operations and in the costs to maintain them. So, although a building's foundations and walls may last for 50 to 100 years, the roof will likely wear out after 20 years and the air-conditioning system in 15 years. The level of maintenance undertaken, the timeliness and quality of the maintenance, the climate, and other factors will also affect the service lives of various systems and components.

Some design changes in green schools may increase the complexity of building systems. No matter how positive the design/engineering and construction gains are for green schools, their ongoing maintenance will be critical to the outcomes for health, learning, and productivity. Thus, the process of creating a green school does not end at the ribbon cutting.

MODELING THE EFFECTS OF GREEN SCHOOLS

Green schools have two complementary, but not identical, goals: (1) to support the development (physical, social, and intellectual) of students, teachers, and staff by providing a healthy, safe, comfortable, and productive physical environment and (2) to have positive environmental and community attributes. Thus, research on green schools might be conceptualized with two quite different sets of outcome measures: improved student and staff health and development, or improved environment and community. In line with its charge, the committee is focusing on outcomes associated with student and teacher health and performance.

An assessment of the outcomes of the quality of a school building on student and teacher health and performance must be set in context. First, time spent in school is, at most, 40 to 50 hours per week, and other environments could equally affect health and performance, including home, neighborhood, recreational, cultural, and religious settings. Even if outcomes could be tied specifically to the quality of the school setting, the influence of other educational factors might be far greater, including quality of curriculum, teacher education/preparation, parental support, peer support, background of student, prior health of student, quality of the administration, and educational standards. For example, research on teaching suggests that student learning is affected by teacher quality (variously defined as teacher experience, teacher knowledge, etc.), and research on learning suggests that student learning may also be affected by the quality of instructional materials, including curriculum, texts, and laboratory equipment. Policy researchers suggest that teaching and learning might be shaped by various state policies regarding teacher education, licensing, hiring, and professional development (Darling-Hammond, 1999), national policies such as the No Child Left Behind Act, and their implementation.

To help inform the committee of mechanisms by which the physical environment might affect student learning, teacher productivity, or the health of students, teachers, and staff, the committee developed a conceptual model for evaluating the research related to such links (Figure 1.1).

---

[2] The annual operation and maintenance costs of a building, however, will be only a fraction of the annual costs to operate an educational institution, which includes the salaries and benefits of teachers, administrators, and support staff; educational equipment and supplies; food service; and other expenses.

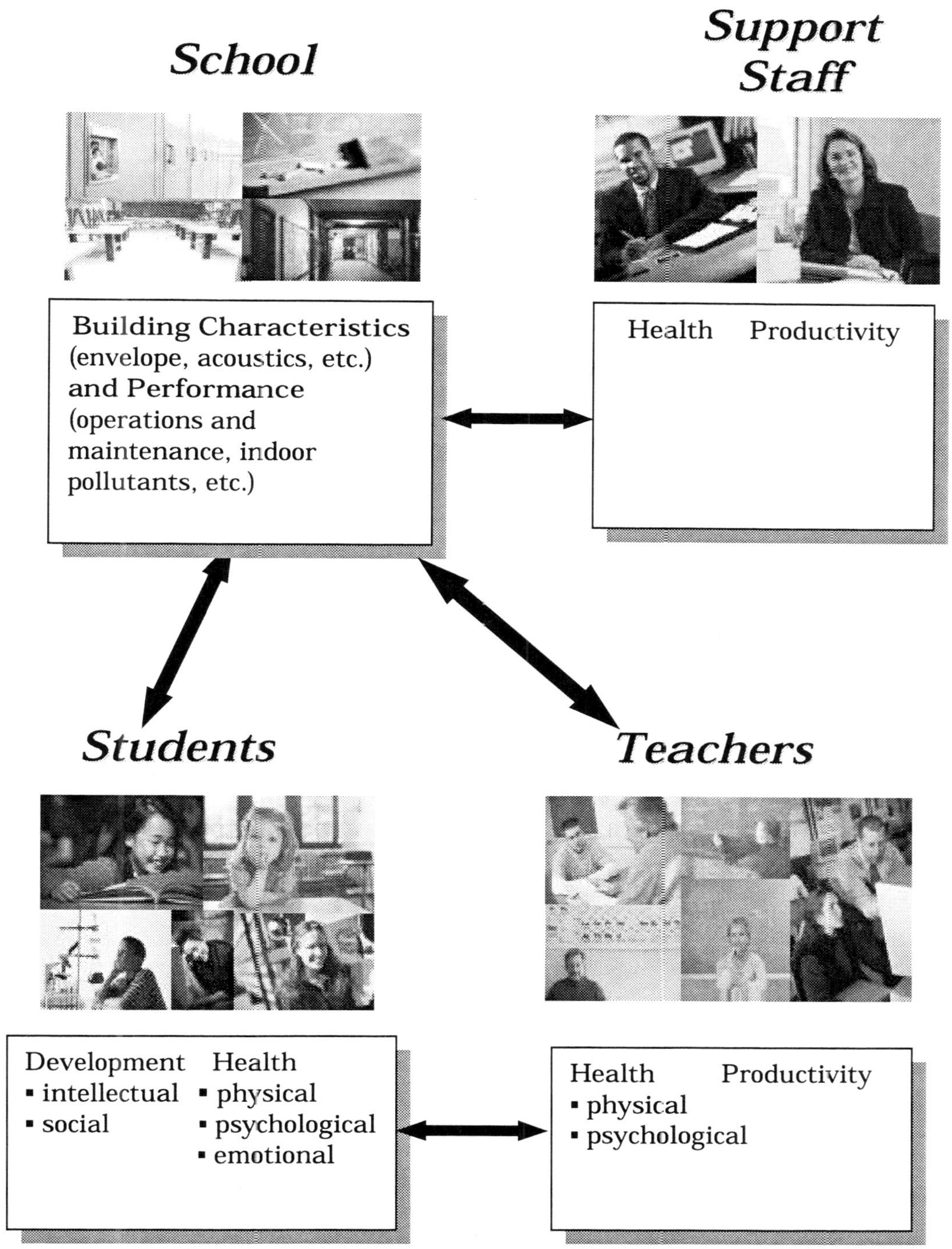

FIGURE 1.1 Conceptual model for evaluating links between school buildings, learning, and health.

School Building Characteristics and Human Response

In the conceptual model, a school building's physical characteristics (envelope, acoustics, lighting) affect an individual by providing an environment with appropriate (or inappropriate) light, sound, temperature, air, spatial condition, and other qualities. The *performance* of a school building and the quality of the environment provided will change by season (e.g., airborne pollen) and over time (e.g., mold growth from chronic water leakage) and will be affected by operational, maintenance, and repair practices and procedures.

Despite the individual nature of systems in school buildings, whether conventional or green, the interactions among systems can determine the overall performance of a building. Ventilation, for example, affects other environmental factors such as temperature, humidity, noise, vibration, and air quality factors of moisture control and microbial contamination. The mechanical ventilation system may also play a role in the transmission of infectious diseases or chemical emissions from materials and products. The location of air intakes, the efficiency of ventilation filters, and the operation of the system all will affect the amount and quality of outdoor air used to ventilate the indoor environment. The quality of a ventilation system's performance will depend on nonmechanical factors such as the level and timeliness of maintenance and repair, the training of maintenance staff, and management and operational practices. How a school is used (for educational purposes only or for community and other activities) and how intensely it is used (9 or 12 months of the year, by how many people) will also affect the overall performance of its systems.

The physical and psychological health of teachers may be affected by a school building's characteristics and conditions. When teachers' well-being suffers, so too might their instruction and their participation in school activities. In that sense, teachers can be seen as both an outcome of building conditions (they might be healthier or not, more motivated or not) and a mediating variable (they might teach differently or interact with students differently depending on their health and well-being) in explaining students' experiences. They may also positively or negatively alter a school's physical setting by adjusting the temperature of a room, opening or closing windows, and other actions.

A second population affected by building characteristics is students. Primary outcomes of interest are student learning and health. Student outcomes might be directly or indirectly related to a school building's condition: If there is high absenteeism at a school among teachers because of poor air quality, the content of instruction may suffer. If students are absent because of poor air quality, there is less opportunity to receive instruction. And, just as teachers can alter the school setting, so too can students.

A third population that can affect and be affected by a school's environment is the administrators (principals, financial staff, counselors, librarians) and support staff (building operations, maintenance, cleaning crews, and kitchen workers). These groups may spend as much time in a school building as teachers and students and sometimes at different times of the day (before and after classes, on weekends, during school breaks and summer vacation). The quality of the support staff training may be of particular significance in the performance of building systems, the timeliness and quality of maintenance and repair, and cleaning and sanitation practices.

Outcomes of Human Responses

It is impossible for researchers to directly access an individual's personal experiences. Instead, access to those experiences is gained indirectly by measuring outcomes such as learning, productivity, or attendance or by revealed preference (surveys). It becomes quite complicated to draw firm inferences about a cause-and-effect relationship between the physical environment and health and performance outcomes for individuals. Often multiple converging lines of research are needed for establishing "scientific fact." In addition, differing populations may have differing responses to features or attributes of the built environment.

In studying the relationships between building characteristics and condition and related teacher and student outcomes, researchers use indicators or surrogates for the relevant variables (Table 1.1). In the studies reviewed by the committee, multiple and quite varied measures were used for both the independent and the dependent variables. One measure, absenteeism, was used as a surrogate measure for student health, teacher health, student learning, and teacher productivity. (The committee plans to discuss outcome indicators in greater detail in its final report.)

TABLE 1.1 Illustrative Example of Indicators Used to Measure Relevant Outcomes

	Student	Teacher
Health	Asthma Allergies Cold/flu and other respiratory diseases Headaches Eye fatigue	Asthma Allergies Cold/flu and other respiratory diseases Vocal fatigue Headaches Eye fatigue
Development (learning and productivity)	Standardized test scores Working memory Prospective memory Sustained attention Reading comprehension Verbal comprehension Demonstration of concepts Graduation rates College enrollment rates Disciplinary incidents	Turnover/retention Attitude/motivation Teaching behaviors/methods Years of experience Knowledge Educational preparation Certification/licensure Teacher examination scores

COMPLEXITY OF THE TASK

The committee has been asked to consider the possible influence of confounding, bias, error, and chance in the relevant literature. Confounding, in particular, poses a major challenge to researchers and those evaluating their work. Confounding occurs when the exposure-adverse event association is biased as a result of a third factor that is capable of causing the adverse event and is statistically associated with the exposure. For example, in any epidemiological study comparing an exposed with a nonexposed group, a simple comparison of the groups may either exaggerate or hide the true difference, because it is likely that the two groups will differ with respect to factors that are also associated with the risk of the outcome of interest, such as socioeconomic status. Said differently, a simple comparison of the incidence of health outcomes among exposed and nonexposed groups may exaggerate an apparent difference because socioeconomic status is also thought to influence the incidence of several health problems.

A variety of confounding factors will be present in any study that attempts to link features of school buildings with student and teacher health and development. Age differences among students will influence the outcomes of research into health and learning: Young children have a higher relative volume of breathing per weight than teenagers; their tissues and organs are actively growing; they are still developing language and cognitive skills; and they spend more time in school than anywhere but home.

Research studies that include the use of any measure of student performance in making comparisons to other variables must try to control extraneous variables that influence the performance of students. For instance, when comparing student achievement test scores with the condition of the physical environment, a researcher would normally attempt to control other influences or variables that affect outcomes. They may include socioeconomic status, the community background of a student or a teacher, or the curriculum. Student test scores will also be influenced by conditions in the classroom on the day of the test and other factors.

Another confounding factor is that school buildings themselves are not standardized, making direct comparisons between school environments problematic. Unlike tract housing developments, most schools are designed by architects as unique structures, whose features depend on the resources available, construction methods, teaching methods, and building codes in effect at the time. They may have one or multiple stories, accommodate a hundred or several thousand students, and may be 5 or 100 years old; all of these factors could potentially influence health and performance outcomes.

The condition of school buildings is also a factor to be considered. School conditions are widely divergent across the country or even within localities. Those school systems with less financial ability and a greater percentage of students from low-income households seem to have school buildings in worse condition than those school systems that have a high tax base and the financial and leadership ability to solve the problems of providing good school buildings for students. Compounding these difficulties is the collection of data about school buildings: The Educational Writers Association (1989) found that few states had sufficient capability to properly evaluate school buildings because the department of education either had few or no personnel to conduct such services. Consequently, the collection of data was erratic.

The Variability and Quality of Research

Gaps in the research literature are also of concern. For example, much of what is known about the impact of the physical environment on health, well-being, and performance is based on studies of adult populations. Some research is quite narrow—in an effort to control for all possible extraneous variables. Other research is so broad that confounding variables are possible, if not likely. In general, much less is known about the impact of the school environment—green or otherwise—on the health and performance of children as compared with the impact of workplace environments on adults. Extrapolating from studies of adults to conclusions about a much younger population can be suspect. For example, environmental factors in the school may interact with genetic factors to determine the degree to which a child develops language skills or displays asthma symptoms. The physical environment could potentially have acute as well as lifelong effects on children's health and performance.

The line of reasoning inherent in this study's task—mapping connections from physical environments to student and teacher outcomes—poses significant challenges concerning cause-and-effect relationships. One challenge is that of directionality of relationships. Green schools might have positive effects on student health, but it might also be that students who live in communities inclined to build green schools are healthier to begin with. Another challenge is that in a conceptual model such as the one used here, the effects of physical environments might be "trumped" in some ways by other forces—teacher quality or parent involvement or financial resources. With outcomes as complex as student health and development—influenced as they are by many school, family, and community factors—it might be impossible to design research that controls for all potentially confounding variables.

A third challenge concerns the variability in the characteristics and standards used by different disciplines to conduct research. For example, medical research may employ clinical trials and intervention studies in which various factors can be controlled for and their results directly evaluated using established protocols. Often clinical trials of drugs include placebos administered according to the same protocol as the drug of interest. Epidemiological studies often rely on statistical significance as a quantitative measure of the extent to which chance or sampling variation might be responsible for an observed association between an exposure and an adverse event. In these studies, quantitative estimation is firmly founded in statistical theory on the basis of repeated sampling.

Studies linking the built environment with the behaviors of its occupants, in contrast, cannot set up strictly controlled trials or easily manipulate variables to test for statistical significance. Studies attempting to link students' and teachers' development with school environments cannot control for the effects of the environments in which students and teachers live during the times when they are in nonschool venues. In addition, there are no standard protocols for conducting building-related research, although some studies have used similar methodologies or evaluation methods, including multiple regression analyses and measures of statistical significance.

Measuring Student Learning and Teacher Productivity

Education is the transferring of knowledge and skills to students and is difficult to measure directly. To measure whether and how well students are learning, indicators or surrogate measures are often used to determine whether cognitive skills are indeed being transferred. Such surrogates include standardized test scores, demonstration of concepts, and graduation rates.

Productivity for an individual or an organization has been defined as the ability to enhance work output through increases in either the quantity and/or the quality of the product or service to be delivered (Boyce et al., 2003). Productivity is influenced both by the individual and the system within which he or she works. Increasing evidence is available to indicate that the built environment can influence both individual and organizational productivity. It can be measured in the number of units manufactured or in the number of words typed correctly in a given amount of time. Absence is often used as a surrogate, the rationale being that people who are absent are less productive than people who are on the job.

For other kinds of work, including teaching, productivity is more difficult to define and measure. Productivity is closely linked to the "quality" of teachers, both individually and collectively. Researchers have used various measures such as years of service, educational preparation, certification/licensure, and scores on teacher examinations (Praxis) in an attempt to obtain a measure of objectivity in determining the quality of the teaching staff. These measures can be quantified to a certain extent and therefore are used quite efficiently in research studies. These measures of quality have not been tested sufficiently, however, to enable a great deal of confidence in their effectiveness. The years of experience a teacher has is to a degree a measure of quality because the teacher is usually evaluated for the decision of granting tenure. To that extent, the quality of the teacher is high enough that the administration decides to retain the teacher because in its judgment the teacher has performed satisfactorily in the years before being considered for tenure. Conversely, there is no guarantee that gaining tenure is anything more than meeting the minimum standards.

For those reasons and because of the multiplicity of variables that can influence learning, evaluations of educational interventions do not often find a significant change in student achievement outcomes. Intensive in-service education for teachers, major revisions of curriculum, and addition of curricular units on substance abuse prevention or economics tend to show small gains at best. Thus, if certain building characteristics or operation practices also are shown to yield only a small gain, at best, in student achievement, such an outcome is not unexpected.

COMMITTEE'S APPROACH

The committee's initial review of the literature focused specifically on those studies that purport to address the connections between sustainable or green building design, student learning and health, and teacher productivity and health. No well-designed, evidence-based studies concerning the overall effects of green schools on the health or development of students and teachers were identified. However, a few studies examined specific building features often emphasized in green school design and the effects of these features on health and performance. Among those are a series of studies on daylighting and student achievement produced by the Heschong-Mahone Group between 1999 and 2003. These studies are discussed in Chapter 4. For the most part, however, the literature on green schools, health, and productivity consists of anecdotal information and case studies of varying quality. The committee also did not identify any evidence-based studies that analyze whether green schools are actually different from conventional schools in regard to the health and productivity of occupants. This lack of well-designed, evidence-based studies specifically related to green schools is understandable, because the concept of green schools is relatively new and evidence-based studies require a significant commitment of time and resources.

A much more robust body of scientific evidence is available that looks at the characteristics emphasized in green school design—building envelope, mechanical and engineering systems, lighting, acoustics—and their relationships to occupant health, development, and productivity. Typically, those studies look at a single system or at a very limited number of variables, and the quality of the studies varies. For example, a literature review of the available evidence on building characteristics, dampness, and health effects identified 590 epidemiological studies addressing these topics. Of these, only 61 met standards for a strong study design and the provision of useful information (NORDAMP, 2002). Relatively few studies look at the interrelationships of two or three building systems and their effects, for example, ventilation, acoustics, learning, and health. With these caveats in mind, the committee determined it should review the scientific literature relating to those characteristics of green schools that are typically emphasized in definitions and guidelines and that differ from conventional school building practices.

However, a review of all research literature that touches on some aspect of buildings and their potential impacts on occupant health, learning, or productivity is an undertaking beyond the resources of this study. In cases in which rigorous reviews of a particular aspect of interest have been conducted by the National Research Council or other organizations or researchers, the committee relies on that work (e.g., IOM, 2004; Mendell and Heath, 2004). In those areas in which the research is fairly limited but important to the study, the committee is conducting its own review. In all cases, the committee describes the source of the literature reviewed, the research methodology used in the studies reviewed, and the basis for the committee's conclusions. Ultimately, the determination of the scope of the literature review must be based on the committee's collective judgment in regard to where its efforts should be concentrated to best address the task statement and meet the sponsors' requirements.

In evaluating the literature, the committee has relied on a hierarchy of evidence for scientific inference developed by the National Academies (Box 1.1) for use in health-related studies (IOM, 1991, 1993, 1994, 1996, 1999, 2003). This hierarchy has played an important role in the committee's deliberations.

Given the level of interaction between people and their environments and other confounding factors, it may never be possible to categorically establish a causal relationship between an attribute of a school building and its effect on students, teachers, and staff. The effects of the built environment will necessarily appear to be small, given the number of variables. Nor may it be possible to quantify the effects of one feature, such as acoustics, on student learning. The committee used its collective best judgment with regard to evaluating the plausibility of the published research and possible explanations of physiological mechanisms, and then integrated the results of those studies found to be useful (if flawed) into its findings, conclusions, and recommendations.

Box 1.1 National Academies' Hierarchy of Evidence for Scientific Inference in Health-Related Studies

Sufficient Evidence of a Causal Relationship: Evidence is sufficient to conclude that a causal relationship exists between the agent and the outcome. That is, the evidence fulfills the criteria for sufficient proof of an association, and in addition, satisfies evaluation criteria such as strength of association, biologic gradient, consistency of association, biologic plausibility and coherence, and temporally correct association. The finding of sufficient evidence of a causal relationship between an exposure and a health outcome does not mean that the exposure would inevitably lead to that outcome. Rather it means that the exposure can cause the outcome, at least in some people under some circumstances.

Sufficient Evidence of an Association: Evidence is sufficient to conclude that there is an association. That is, an association between the agent and the outcome has been observed in studies in which chance, bias, and confounding can be ruled out with reasonable confidence.

Limited or Suggestive Evidence of an Association: Evidence is suggestive of an association between the agent and the outcome but is limited because chance, bias, and confounding could not be ruled out with confidence. For example, at least one high-quality study shows a positive association, but the results of other studies are inconsistent.

Inadequate or Insufficient Evidence to Determine Whether or Not an Association Exists: The available studies are of insufficient quality, consistency, or statistical power to permit a conclusion about the presence or absence of an association. Alternatively, no studies exist that examine the relationship.

Limited or Suggestive Evidence of No Association: Several adequate studies are consistent in not showing an association between the agent and the outcome. A conclusion of "no association" is inevitably limited to the conditions, magnitude of exposure, and length of observation covered by the available studies.

SOURCE: IOM, 2004.

Empirical measures do not, however, necessarily capture all relevant considerations that should be applied when evaluating research results. Qualitative aspects of the environment are also important. Thus, in the committee's collective judgment, there is value in attempting to identify design features and building processes and practices that may lead to improvements in learning, health, and productivity for students, teachers, and other school staff, even if empirical results are less than robust.

Chapters 2 through 6 of this interim report present the committee's findings and recommendations related to building envelope, moisture management, and health; ventilation, pollutant source control, health, and productivity; lighting, performance, and health; acoustics, student learning, and teacher health; and building condition and student achievement. As noted previously, additional topic areas, findings, and recommendations will be included in the committee's final report.

FINDINGS

Finding 1: In its review thus far, the committee has found the following:

- There are no well-designed, evidence-based studies concerning the overall effects of green schools on the health or development of students and teachers, in part because the concept of green schools is quite new. There are, however, a few well-designed studies that examine specific building features often emphasized in green school design and the effects of these components on health and learning.
- Given the level of interaction between people and their environments and other confounding factors, establishing cause-and-effect relationships between an attribute of a school building and its effect on students, teachers, and staff is difficult. The effects of the built environment will necessarily appear to be small, given the number of variables.
- Empirical measures do not, however, necessarily capture all relevant considerations that should be applied when evaluating research results. Qualitative aspects of the environment are also important. Thus, in the committee's collective judgment, there is value in attempting to identify design features and building processes and practices that may lead to improvements in learning, health, and productivity for students, teachers, and other school staff, even if empirical results are less than robust.

2

Building Envelope, Moisture Management, and Health

The foundation, walls, windows, and roof of a building make up an "envelope" intended to shelter people and equipment from the weather, and from natural and man-made hazards. Windows and doors allow outside air, light, people, equipment, and supplies to enter or exit a building. Skylights allow in daylight. Building envelopes can be designed for natural ventilation or for mechanically conditioned air or hybrid systems. Whether planned or not, buildings have openings that allow the penetration and internal movement of air, water, and contaminants.

Typically, guidelines for green schools address building envelope issues concerning siting, glazing, natural ventilation, and materials. Typically, the conservation of water, both outside and inside the building, is addressed through landscaping-related efforts such as irrigation, and plumbing-related features, such as restrooms. Existing guidelines are silent for the most part about building envelope per se except in reference to roofs and sound attenuation of outside noise. The committee believes that the design, construction, and maintenance of the building envelope are critical to green schools and therefore should have a more prominent place in any set of green school guidelines, for the reasons outlined below.

BUILDING ENVELOPE AND MOISTURE MANAGEMENT

It is popularly thought that green buildings are those buildings that are constructed using specific materials, systems, and technologies. However, it may not be as obvious that "dry" is a primary design objective for a green school building. Moisture ranks as a leading cause of structural damage, and excess moisture in a building has been associated with a variety of health problems in children and adults (IOM, 2004).

Water-related issues in buildings originate from many sources: groundwater, plumbing failures, construction materials, occupants, and the external environment. As long as a building is properly designed, sited, constructed, operated, and maintained, water can be managed effectively. However, excess water or moisture in a building can lead to structural failures and health-related problems when materials stay wet long enough for microbial growth, physical deterioration, or chemical reactions to occur (IOM, 2004). A complex set of moisture-transport processes related to climate, building design, construction, operation, and maintenance determine whether a building will have a moisture problem that could influence the health of the occupants.

Well-designed moisture control considers the potential damage and degree of risk associated with each of the following four transport mechanisms (from most to least potent):

1. Bulk transport,
2. Capillary transport,

3. Air transport, and
4. Vapor diffusion.

Bulk transport, or leakage of rain, melting snow, and groundwater through the building envelope, is orders of magnitude more destructive than any other force. Capillary movement of water from the outside of the building into the building through porous surfaces and the movement of air-transported water vapor are second and third in the rank order of transport mechanisms. Both represent a significant threat and require dedicated attention during design and construction. Vapor diffusion is a relatively weak force but also requires careful detailing and execution of building assemblies. Excellent resources for proper moisture control design include *The Moisture Control Handbook, Principles and Practices for Residential and Small Commercial Buildings* by Joseph Lstiburek and John Carmody (1994) and *The Building Foundation Design Handbook* (ORNL, 1988).

EXCESSIVE MOISTURE AND HEALTH

Recently there has been concern that indoor moisture "dampness" and mold growth can lead to a variety of health problems in adults and children. The most consistent and convincing associations relate to respiratory disease, especially asthma. Asthma is a disorder of airflow obstruction. People with asthma are subject to episodic wheezing, coughing, and shortness of breath. Although these symptoms are common clinical features of asthma, they are common symptoms of other respiratory illnesses as well. Finding a widely accepted definition of this disease has proved problematic, and the following has been offered as the most acceptable:

> Asthma is understood to be a chronic disease of the airways characterized by an inflammatory response involving many cell types. Both genetic and environmental factors appear to play important roles in the initiation and continuation of the inflammation. Although the inflammatory response may vary from one patient to another, the symptoms are often episodic and usually include wheezing, breathlessness, chest tightness, and coughing. Symptoms may occur at any time of the day, but are more commonly seen at night. These symptoms are associated with widespread airflow obstruction that is at least partially reversible with pharmacologic agent or time. Many persons with asthma also have varying degrees of bronchial hyperresponsiveness. Research has shown that after long periods of time this inflammation may cause a gradual alteration or remodeling of the architecture of the lungs that cannot be reversed with therapy. (IOM, 2000, pp. 23-24)

Asthma affects 8 percent to 10 percent of the population and even larger proportions of children in certain cities or poor urban populations. It is a common reason that children are absent from school and one of the most common causes of work absences as well; 14 million days of school loss were recorded in 1994-1996, 3.4 days per child with asthma (Cox-Ganser et al., 2005).

Indoor environments are an important factor in chronic asthma symptoms and morbidity, whether these environments are in the home or in the school. The Institute of

Medicine (IOM) has issued two reports on the association of excessive moisture or "dampness," mold growth, and respiratory illness in building occupants, *Clearing the Air: Asthma and Indoor Air Exposures* (IOM, 2000) and *Damp Indoor Spaces and Health* (IOM, 2004). Both concluded that damp, moldy buildings were associated with respiratory symptoms both in people with asthma and in the general population. To the extent that they might affect indoor dampness, green school designs might affect students' health and productivity. If school buildings can be designed to minimize the contribution to asthma morbidity, they can have a positive impact on health and performance.

The report *Damp Indoor Spaces and Health* considered separately the common respiratory symptoms (wheeze, cough, shortness of breath) and the diagnosis of asthma (usually based on reported physician diagnosis, reversible obstruction measured by lung function tests, or use of appropriate medication by the respondent). In addition, the report distinguished asthma development (the appearance of asthma for the first time) from asthma exacerbations (asthma symptoms in persons with a diagnosis of chronic asthma).

Using the National Academies' hierarchy of evidence for scientific inference (see Box 1.1), the report found *sufficient evidence of an association* between indoor dampness and several respiratory health outcomes, although the evidence was not strong enough to say there was a causal relationship. In the case of asthma, the association was found in people with asthma in general.

There are at least two distinct variants of asthma: an extrinsic, allergic variant that occurs in the context of immunoglobulin E (IgE)-mediated sensitization to environmental allergens and an intrinsic, nonallergic variant with no detectable sensitization and low IgE concentrations. In both variants, the airways are strikingly hyperresponsive, and symptoms may also be mediated by irritant responses. In those studies that evaluated asthmatic patients for IgE-mediated sensitization, the association was stronger in sensitized individuals; thus the IOM study concluded that the association was strongest in sensitized individuals. In addition, an association between dampness and mold and the symptoms of cough or wheeze was consistently found in studies of the general population. Because asthma has been diagnosed in only 8 percent to 10 percent of the population, it was unlikely that this relationship could be accounted for in these studies by asthma alone. Thus, the 2004 IOM study concluded that moisture and mold were associated with cough and wheeze in the general population.

The existing evidence was considered to be insufficient to support an association between dampness and mold and asthma *development* because fewer studies were available. Of the 10 studies available, only 1 (Jaakola et al., 2002) found that the association was insignificant. The others found an association with moisture, mold, or both. Particularly important were the three birth cohort studies (Belanger et al., 2003; Slezak et al., 1998; Maier et al., 1997) in which infants and children who were genetically at risk to develop asthma were observed for several years. Stark et al. (2003) reported on a birth cohort of 849 infants less than 1 year old who had at least one sibling with physician-diagnosed asthma; they found that wheeze and persistent cough were associated with measured airborne concentrations of *Penicillium* and *Cladosporium*, two types of mold commonly found in indoor air samples.

Finally, upper respiratory symptoms (nasal congestion, sneezing, runny or itchy nose) were associated with damp indoor environments and mold. Like asthma, chronic rhinitis has an allergic and a nonallergic variant. The allergic variant occurs in the context of IgE-mediated sensitization to environmental allergens. In the studies included in the 2004 IOM report, upper respiratory symptoms were associated with dampness and mold in persons with self-identified allergic rhinitis, as well as in the general population. Other studies reported that the frequency of "colds," that is, acute viral infectious rhinitis, was associated with dampness and mold. Because the cause of upper respiratory symptoms could not be identified, the committee concluded that the symptoms, but not a specific illness, were associated.

The mechanisms by which damp indoor spaces and mold are associated with respiratory illness are not clear, but there are several possibilities. First, many people with asthma demonstrate IgE-mediated sensitization to mold, so the possibility exists that symptoms are related to specific immune mechanisms. Mold produces a number of materials such as peptidoglycans and polysaccharides that induce inflammation through the innate immune pathways; other materials such as volatile organic compounds[3] and toxins may have direct effects because asthmatic airways have a characteristic hyperresponsiveness and are excessively responsive to exposures to irritants. Other organisms such as gram-negative or gram-positive bacteria might coexist with mold in damp environments; endotoxin or lipoteichoic acid from these organisms might induce airway symptoms. Finally, the interaction of moisture and mold with building materials may produce metabolites that have direct irritant effects on asthmatic airways. The multiplicity of possible mechanisms illustrates that the pathways to respiratory effects will be complex, but all of these mechanisms are plausible consequences of excessive indoor moisture. Maintaining structures that are dry (i.e., without excessive moisture) potentially could prevent all of these effects.

The findings of key relevance to this interim report from *Damp Indoor Spaces and Health* are summarized in Box 2.1.

---

[3] Volatile organic compounds (VOCs) are emitted as gases from certain solids or liquids. VOCs include a variety of chemicals, some of which may have short- and long-term adverse health effects.

Box 2.1 Findings from the Institute of Medicine Relevant to This Study

Sufficient Evidence of an Association Between Dampness and Respiratory Health

- Asthma symptoms in sensitized persons
- Cough
- Wheeze
- Upper respiratory (nasal and throat) tract symptoms

Limited or Suggestive Evidence of an Association

- Asthma development
- Dyspnea (shortness of breath)
- Lower respiratory illness in otherwise healthy children

Sufficient Evidence of an Association Between Mold or Other Agents and Respiratory Health

- Asthma symptoms in sensitized persons
- Cough
- Wheeze
- Upper respiratory (nose and throat) tract symptoms
- Hypersensitivity pneumonitis in susceptible individuals

Limited or Suggestive Evidence of an Association

- Lower respiratory illness in otherwise healthy children

SOURCE: IOM, 2004.

In addition to potential health benefits, designing for effective moisture management will likely have benefits for the building as well. The more durable a building is, the longer its components will last (Deal et al., 1998). The materials in long-lived building assemblies are replaced less frequently than in nondurable structures. This makes dry structures resource and energy efficient, because new replacement materials are not harvested, mined, and produced, nor is energy used to make, transport, and assemble the replacement components. Dry buildings also require fewer resources and money to repair and maintain. For example, damp surfaces cause stains and peeling paint that require frequent repainting and cleaning. For these reasons, dry buildings may have lower life-cycle costs associated with them.

FINDINGS AND RECOMMENDATION

Finding 2: In regard to issues related to building envelope, moisture management, and health, the committee has found the following:

- There is sufficient evidence to establish an association between moisture problems in buildings (floods, visible dampness, leaks, mold growth in spaces or in heating, ventilation, and air-conditioning [HVAC] systems) and adverse health outcomes, particularly asthma and respiratory symptoms, among children and adults.
- Excessive moisture in a building can lead to structural damage, deterioration of the performance of building systems and components, and cosmetic damage, all of which can result in increased maintenance and repair costs.
- Guidelines for green schools typically do not adequately address the design detailing, construction, and long-term maintenance of building envelopes to ensure that allergen sources are controlled, moisture is controlled, and a building is kept dry over the long term.
- Well-designed, constructed, and maintained building envelopes are critical to the control and prevention of the excessive moisture and molds that have been associated with adverse health effects in children and adults Designing for effective moisture management will likely have benefits for the building, including lower life-cycle costs. Excellent resources for proper moisture control design include *The Moisture Control Handbook, Principles and Practices for Residential and Small Commercial Buildings* by Joseph Lstiburek and John Carmody (1994) and *The Building Foundation Design Handbook* (ORNL, 1988).

Recommendation 1: The control of excessive moisture, dampness, and molds to protect the health of children and adults in schools and to protect the structural integrity of a building should be a key objective for green schools. MASSTECH should develop guidelines that specifically address moisture control as it relates to the design, construction, operation, and maintenance of a school building's envelope (foundations, walls, windows, and roofs) and ventilation systems, and related items such as siting, landscaping, and plumbing systems.

3

Ventilation, Pollutant Source Control, Health, and Performance

The primary purpose of a building's heating, ventilation, and air-conditioning (HVAC) system is to provide comfort for the occupants by meeting thermal requirements and diluting contaminants. HVAC systems accomplish this through the conditioning of outside air coming into occupied spaces and the removal of irritants and pollutants. The principal standards and guidelines for HVAC system design and operation include (1) American Society of Heating, Refrigeration, and Air Conditioning Engineers (ASHRAE) Standard 62.1-2004, "Ventilation for Acceptable Indoor Air Quality"; (2) American National Standards Institute (ANSI)/ASHRAE Standard 55-2004, "Thermal Environmental Conditions for Human Occupancy"; (3) the Department of Energy EnergySmart Schools guidelines; and (4) individual state codes, some of which are based on or reference other codes such as the International Building Code.

Green school guidelines typically address HVAC systems as they relate to energy efficiency, indoor air quality (ventilation), moisture control, filter efficiencies and maintenance, and the elimination of CFC-based refrigerants.

In a comprehensive review of the literature related to indoor air quality, ventilation, and health symptoms in schools, Daisey et al. (2003) found the following:

- Reported ventilation and carbon dioxide (CO_2) levels indicated that a significant proportion of classrooms did not meet the (then) ASHRAE standard 62-1999 for minimum ventilation rate;[4]
- A variety of volatile organic compounds (VOCs) and bioaerosols (primarily molds and fungi, dust mites, and animal antigens) could be found in school environments; and
- Although there were a number of studies in which typical building-related symptoms[5] were measured, there was a relative paucity of literature in which specific building conditions or measured pollutants were then linked to specific symptoms.

The following sections address some aspects of indoor air quality and pollutant source control, ventilation rates, and moisture management in HVAC systems. The committee plans to address additional issues related to HVAC systems, including temperature and humidity, in its final report.

---

[4] The ASHRAE standard has since been revised.

[5] Building-related symptoms, frequently referred to as "sick building syndrome," have been defined as a set of symptoms reported subjectively by occupants of a building that may improve when they leave the building. Symptoms include eye, nose, and throat irritations; headaches; fatigue; difficulty breathing; itching; and dry, irritated skin (FFC, 2005).

INDOOR AIR QUALITY AND POLLUTANT SOURCE CONTROL

There are many sources of exposure to pollutants internal and external to a school. Internal sources include stationary and (potentially) mobile combustion sources; building materials and equipment; educational materials; cleaning products; biological agents; and human activity. External sources include combustion sources (stationary and mobile); biological material; and soil gases (e.g., radon, VOCs from municipal waste sites) particulate matter, and ozone entering through air intakes and the building envelope.

Outdoor Sources

Outdoor sources of air pollution can affect the health of children and adults in two ways. First, students, teachers, and administrative and support staff are exposed to outdoor pollutants before they enter a building, which can lead to increased respiratory symptoms (Schwartz, 2004). Second, outdoor sources of pollution can contribute to indoor air pollutant concentrations through several routes: outdoor air is drawn into a school building by the ventilation system through air intakes located at the rooftop, at ground level, or from below-grade "wells." Outside air also enters the building through doors and windows and through leaks in the building envelope. People themselves can carry viruses, bacteria, pollen, and pollutants, such as dust mites and pet dander, into a school on their shoes and clothing.

Mendell and Heath (2004) found that "a substantial literature of strongly designed cohort studies is available on associations between outdoor pollutants and attendance of children at school" (p. 9). They concluded that there was strongly suggestive evidence that absence from school increased with exposure to ozone at higher concentrations. However, the findings were mixed on associations of school absence with exposure to outdoor nitrogen oxides, carbon dioxide, and particles $<10\ \mu$ in aerodynamic diameter.

Pollen Exposure

Other significant sources of pollutants outside schools are plant-derived materials, or biomass, which can generate bioaerosols, including molds, fungi, and pollen. The 2000 IOM study *Clearing the Air* found as follows:

> Although there is sufficient evidence to conclude that pollen exposure is associated with exacerbation of existing asthma in sensitized individuals, and pollen allergens have been documented in both dust and indoor air, there is inadequate or insufficient information to determine whether indoor air exposure to pollen is associated with exacerbation of asthma. (p. 8)

The study also noted that "there is relatively little information on the impact of ventilation and air cleaning measures on indoor pollen levels, although it is clear that shutting windows and other measures that limit the entry rate of unfiltered air can be effective" (p. 14).

Indoor Sources

There are numerous pollutants in a school building. These pollutants include particulate matter, chemicals, and biological particles or organisms. Sources include building materials (e.g., structural materials such as particleboard, adhesives, insulation); furnishings (carpets, paints, furniture); products used in the building (cleaning materials, pesticides, markers, art supplies); and in some cases the occupants themselves (CO_2, pet hair).

There are a limited number of studies in which source reduction or control methods in schools have been related to pollutant exposures. Smedje and Norbäck (2001) observed that classrooms with more frequent cleaning had lower concentrations of cat and dog antigen in settled dust. However, few studies have looked systematically at changes in exposure, health effects, or productivity based on changes in building materials or products used in schools.

The literature on source reduction and control in homes, particularly with asthmatic children, is more extensive (Takaro et al., 2004). Integrated pest management techniques have been shown to be effective in reducing antigen levels in homes (Phipatanakul et al., 2004) and have been shown to reduce pesticide levels in schools (Williams et al., 2005). However, whether they result in better health outcomes or productivity in schools has not been determined (Phipatanakul et al., 2004; Williams et al., 2005). A recent review by Shendell and others (2004a) examined the various sources and types of controls available for these sources. The committee will address those issues in greater detail in its final report.

INDOOR AIR QUALITY AND VENTILATION RATES

Ventilation rate is based on the outdoor air requirements of a ventilation system. A number of studies have reviewed the effect of ventilation rates on health, productivity, and airborne pollutant control. Although the majority of these studies have been in environments other than schools, there have been several more recent studies and reviews either specifically on schools or including schools in the overall study. Typically, these studies also look at a second variable, such as temperature or humidity, components of thermal comfort, to identify any confounding or synergistic effects.

School-Related Studies

Mendell and Heath (2004) looked at the literature and found

- Suggestive, although not fully consistent, evidence linking low outdoor ventilation rates in buildings to decreased performance in children and adults, and
- Suggestive but inconsistent evidence linking lower ventilation rates with decreased attendance among adults.

Wargocki et al. (2005) conducted a field intervention experiment in two classes of 10-year-old children. Average air temperatures were reduced from 23.6°C to 20°C, and outdoor air supply rates were increased from 5.2 to 9.6 liters per second (l/s) per person in a 2 x 2 crossover design, each condition lasting a week. Tasks representing eight different aspects of schoolwork, from reading to mathematics, were performed during appropriate lessons, and the children marked visual-analogue scales each week to indicate building-related symptom intensity. Increased ventilation rate increased work rate in addition, multiplication, number checking ($p < .05$), and subtraction ($p < .06$). Reduced temperature increased work rate in subtraction and reading ($p < .001$), and reduced errors in checking a transcript against a recorded voice reading aloud ($p < .07$). Reduced temperature at increased ventilation rate increased work rate in a test of logical thinking ($p < .03$). Their experimental data indicated that increasing ventilation rates from 5.4 to 9.6 l/s per person and decreasing temperatures from 24°C to 20°C potentially would improve the performance of schoolwork by children.

Smedje et al. (2000) investigated the impact of improving the ventilation systems in schools on allergies, asthma, and asthma symptoms in schoolchildren. They issued questionnaires to 1,476 children in 39 schools (mixed primary and secondary schools) during the 1993-1995 period. Various exposure factors were measured during this time period in 100 classrooms. In 12 percent of the classrooms, new ventilation systems were installed, increasing the air-exchange rate and reducing the humidity levels in the schools. The air pollutant levels in these schools were lowered with the installation of the new ventilation systems as compared with the levels in the classrooms without the new ventilation systems. Also, the incidence of asthma symptoms, but not allergies, was reduced in the classrooms with the new ventilation systems. Their results indicated an improvement in the children's health in the classrooms with increased ventilation, lower humidity levels, and reduced airborne pollutant levels.

Shendell et al. (2004b) explored the association between student absences and indoor CO_2 levels. These researchers noted that "since measuring the actual ventilation rate is expensive and potentially problematic, the indoor concentration of carbon dioxide (CO_2) has often been used as a surrogate for the ventilation rate per occupant, including in schools." They measured the short-term (5 min) CO_2 levels in 409 traditional and 25 portable classrooms from 22 schools in Washington state. Attendance data were collected from school records. Their results indicated that a 1,000-ppm increase above the outdoor concentration of CO_2 was associated with statistically significant 10 percent to 20 percent increases in student absences. Although student absences are not a direct measurement of student performance, an increased number of absences may contribute to poorer student performance.

Studies of Offices and Other Building Types

In a study of 3,720 hourly employees of a large Massachusetts manufacturer in 40 buildings with 115 independently ventilated working areas, Milton et al. (2000) analyzed the relationship between the rate at which outdoor air was supplied for ventilation and the amount of sick leave taken. The researchers found "consistent associations of increased sick leave with lower levels of outdoor air supply and IEQ [indoor environmental quality] complaints" (p. 212). Seppanen and Fisk (2004) further developed a quantitative relationship by fitting the data from these epidemiological studies by using the Wells-Riley model of airborne disease transmission to predict the relationship. The model predicted that there would be a decrease in illness over time with increasing ventilation rates.

Seppanen et al. (1999) reviewed the literature on the association of ventilation rates in nonresidential and nonindustrial buildings (primarily offices) with health and performance outcomes. The review included 20 studies investigating the association of ventilation rates with human responses and 21 studies investigating the association of CO_2 levels with human responses. A majority of studies found that ventilation rates of less than 10 l/s per person were associated in all building types with a statistically significant worsening in one or more health or perceived air quality outcomes. Some studies found that increasing ventilation rates up to 20 l/s per person was associated with significant decreases in the prevalence of building-related symptoms or with further significant improvements in perceived air quality. The ventilation rate studies reported relative risks of 1.1 to 6 for building-related symptoms for low compared to high ventilation rates.

VENTILATION AND HEALTH

Ventilation and health in nonindustrial indoor environments were the subjects of a European Multidisciplinary Scientific Consensus Meeting (EUROVEN) review of the scientific literature on the effects of ventilation on health, comfort, and productivity in offices, schools, homes, and other nonindustrial environments (Wargocki et al., 2002). The group reviewed 105 papers and judged 30 as being conclusive, providing sufficient evidence on ventilation, health effects, data processing, and reporting. The EUROVEN group agreed that ventilation is strongly associated with comfort (perceived air quality) and health (building-related symptoms, inflammation, infections, asthma, allergy, short-term sick leave) and found an association between ventilation and productivity (performance of office work). They concluded that increasing outdoor air supply rates in nonindustrial environments improves the perceived air quality, and that outdoor air supply rates of less than 25 l/s per person increase the risk of building-related symptoms, increase short-term sick leave, and decrease productivity among occupants of office buildings.

Seppanen and Fisk (2005) reviewed the scientific literature regarding the effects of ventilation on indoor air quality and health, focusing on office-type buildings. Overall their literature review indicated that ventilation has a significant impact on several important user outcomes, including:

- Communicable respiratory illnesses,
- Building-related symptoms,
- Task performance and productivity,
- Perceived air quality among occupants and sensory panels, and
- Respiratory allergies and asthma.

The literature review also indicated that better hygiene, commissioning, operation, and maintenance of air handling systems may be particularly important for reducing the negative effects of HVAC systems. Ventilation may also have harmful effects on indoor air quality and climate if not properly designed, installed, maintained, and operated. The committee will address the literature on ventilation and health in greater detail in its final report.

VENTILATION AND COMFORT

Fang et al. (1998) and Toftum et al. (1998) showed that perceived air quality is strongly influenced by the humidity and the temperature of inhaled air even when the chemical composition of the air is constant and the thermal sensation for the entire body is kept neutral. These findings address the importance of the second purpose of ventilation systems, which is to condition the air to comfortable levels of temperature and humidity. There is a robust literature on the effects of temperature and humidity on both comfort and productivity, although it is based primarily on studies in office buildings (Fanger, 2000; Seppanen and Fisk, 2005; Wyon, 2004). Studies show that productivity declines if temperatures go too high (Federspiel et al., 2004). The committee will address the literature on temperature, health, and performance in greater detail in its final report.

Quantifying Relationships Among Ventilation, Health, and Productivity

Although there is good evidence that HVAC system characteristics can and do affect occupant health and comfort, including in schools, until recently there have been few studies that attempted to measure the magnitude of either the health or productivity effects. Several recent reviews, however, have attempted to quantify the relationship of ventilation rate and pollutant transport to the health and productivity of people indoors.

Wyon (2004) investigated the productivity of office workers based on reducing indoor air pollutant loads by source removal or increasing ventilation rate. Wyon showed that during realistic experimental exposures lasting up to 5 hours, the performance of simulated office work was significantly increased (by approximately 6 percent to 9 percent) by the removal of common indoor sources of air pollution, such as floor-coverings, old supply air filters, and personal computers, or by keeping the sources in place while increasing the clean air ventilation rate from 3 to 30 l/s per person. Wyon then went on to confirm these laboratory findings in a field investigation during an 8-week period. A reduction in pollutant loads in buildings can be expected to reduce building-related symptoms.

Seppanen and Fisk (2005) used previous studies (primarily in office buildings) to develop a model relating building ventilation rates, perceived air quality, and temperature to occupant symptoms and productivity. They estimated that increasing the average ventilation rate from 0.45 to 1.0 exchanges per hour would decrease the sick leave prevalence in an office from 2 percent (5 days per year) to 1.6 percent (3.9 days per year).

MOISTURE MANAGEMENT IN HEATING, VENTILATION, AND AIR-CONDITIONING SYSTEMS

Several findings in the 2004 IOM study *Damp Indoor Spaces and Health* pertain specifically to the design and operation of HVAC systems as a critical factor in the control of moisture in buildings:

- Although relatively little attention has been directed to dampness and mold growth in HVAC systems, there is evidence of associated health effects (p. 42).

- Liquid water is often present at several locations in or near commercial-building HVAC systems, facilitating the growth of microorganisms that may contribute to symptoms or illnesses (p. 42).
- Microbial contamination of HVAC systems has been reported in many case studies and investigated in a few multibuilding efforts (p. 43).
- Sites of reported contamination include outside air louvers, mixing boxes (where outside air mixes with recirculated air), filters, cooling coils, cooling coil drain pans, humidifiers, and duct surfaces (p. 43).
- Bioaerosols from contaminated sites in an HVAC system may be transported to occupants and deposited on previously clean surfaces, making microbial contamination of HVAC systems a potential risk factor for adverse health effects (p. 43).
- Menzies study of ultraviolet germicidal radiation of drip pans and cooling coils shows that limiting microbial contamination of HVAC systems may yield health benefits, and follow-up research is recommended (p. 44).

In addition to moisture and mold, other allergens and irritants found in school buildings may affect a substantial minority of students, teachers, and staff through the same pathways described above. Indoor environments contain varying quantities of allergens from a variety of sources: house dust mites, cat and dog dander, cockroaches, rodents, and seasonal pollens. Indoor concentrations of particulates and various gaseous pollutants (ozone, NO_2, VOCs) may be higher than those found in outside air. The strength of the association of each of these agents was summarized in *Clearing the Air: Asthma and Indoor Air Exposures* (IOM, 2000), and many of them were found to be more strongly related to asthmatic symptoms than were moisture and mold. Through proper design and maintenance practices, green schools can minimize the effects of these exposures. This may involve simple measures such as closing the windows during pollen season or prohibiting furry pets in a school. In other cases, more subtle design considerations may be needed, for example, limiting food preparation, vending, and eating to certain areas with structural and finish features that allow easy pest control.

Taken together, these findings indicate the significant role that HVAC system design and operation play in controlling moisture and pollutants inside buildings.

FINDINGS

Finding 3: In regard to ventilation, pollutant source control, health, and performance, the committee has found the following:

- Numerous pollution sources and building system characteristics affect air quality in a school. The most important determinants of indoor air quality are (1) design and operation of the ventilation system to limit the buildup of pollutants and humidity and achieve thermal comfort, (2) control of indoor sources of pollutants, and (3) control of outdoor sources of pollutants.
- There is a robust body of evidence indicating that the health of children and adults can be affected by air quality in a school.

- A growing body of evidence suggests that teacher productivity and student learning, as measured by absenteeism, may be affected by indoor air quality as well.
- Indoor pollutants and allergens from house dust mites, pet dander, cockroaches, and rodents also contribute to increased respiratory and asthma symptoms among children and adults.
- The reduction of pollutant loads, both sensory and not, has been shown to reduce the occurrence of building-associated symptoms and to improve the health and comfort of people occupying the buildings.
- Although compliance with the American Society for Heating, Refrigeration, and Air-Conditioning Engineers (ASHRAE) standards for ventilation rates may be the minimal acceptable standard for green schools, there is good evidence that increasing the ventilation rate beyond the ASHRAE standard will further improve comfort and productivity. However, an upper limit on the ventilation rates, indicating when the benefits of outside air begin to decline, has not been established.

The committee will address additional issues related to heating, ventilation, and air-conditioning systems and their associations with health and productivity in its final report. Until this review is completed and the results are synthesized, the committee will defer making specific recommendations.

4

Lighting, Performance, and Health

Typically, when addressing lighting requirements, guidelines for green schools focus on energy-efficient lighting systems and the use of daylighting to further conserve energy. They also encourage access to views through the installation of windows.

For purposes of learning, performance, and productivity, lighting in a school building should allow people to see to read, to see others with whom they are communicating, and to perform other visual tasks associated with learning, teaching, and school administration. Lighting can be provided by electric sources or by daylight through windows, clerestories, and skylights Typically, school buildings use a combination of electric lighting and daylight.

Electric lighting systems are made up of a series of components: luminaires, lamps (incandescent, fluorescent, high-intensity discharge [HID]), ballasts (except when using incandescent lamps), and controls. Electric lighting systems differ in the amount of power they require to operate and in the amount and direction of light they are able to generate for the design objectives. They also vary in their initial cost, ease of maintenance and commissioning, and expected life. Also important, electric lighting systems vary in their ability to provide good color rendering, low glare, low flicker, and low noise.

Fluorescent lighting systems are the most prevalent sources of general illumination in schools. Modern fluorescent systems (T8 and T5 lamps with electronic ballasts) can provide low cost, long life, high efficacy, good color, low noise, and low flicker. Other sources of illumination, including incandescent and HID, can be specified in schools to best accomplish specific design objectives, from outdoor applications such as sports fields to illuminating pictures or works of art (Rea and Bullough, 2001).

Windows are an important part of the school design.[6] First and foremost, windows provide a view to the outside. They also provide high light levels and, when properly located, ideal eye-task-lighting geometries for reflective visual tasks (i.e., those other than self-luminous displays, such as computer screens, and audio visual presentations). Skylights and clerestories can also be beneficial sources of illumination even though they do not provide a view.

A key difference between designs with electric light and/or daylight is that electric light is almost always static, whereas daylight is ever changing over the course of a day, with weather conditions, and with season. Daylight will also be different from one school to another, depending on building orientation and site, local climate, and latitude, so a “cookie cutter” building design will rarely provide ideal lighting conditions. The dynamic nature of daylight, together with its wide range of intensities and geometries, demands a dedicated understanding of its interactions with the building and its spaces. In some circumstances it may be desirable to conduct detailed lighting, heating, and cooling simulations in order to gain such an understanding. The potential benefits of higher lighting levels, excellent color

[6] This discussion is restricted to the lighting effects of windows.

and form rendition, views, and the temporal lighting qualities may justify this careful design requirement and additional analyses.

LIGHTING AND ITS IMPACT ON THE VISUAL AND CIRCADIAN SYSTEMS

When evaluating the performance of any lighting system, electric or daylight, its impact on two biological systems—the visual and the circadian—needs to be considered together with the physical attributes of light that differentially affect these systems (Figure 4.1).

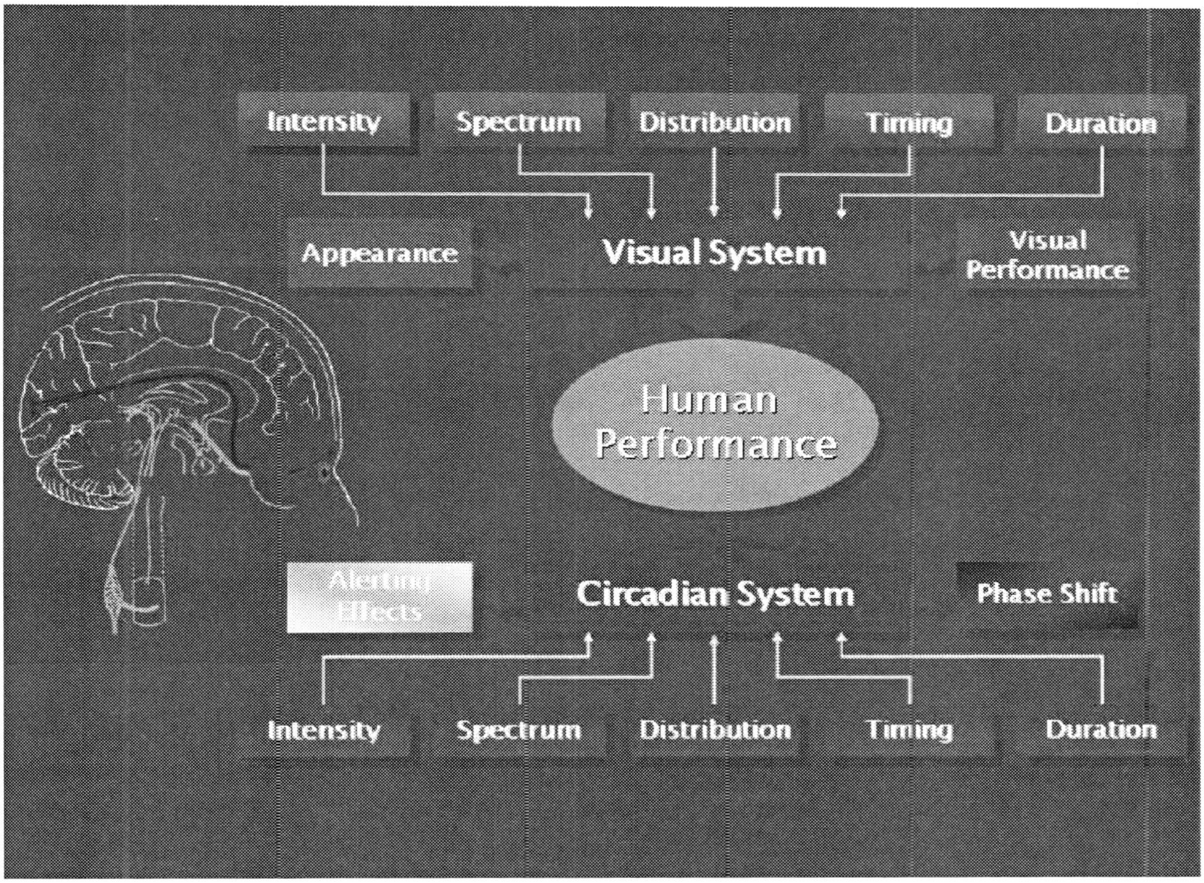

FIGURE 4.1 Light as it affects human performance and health through the visual and circadian systems. SOURCE: Lighting Research Center.

The Visual System

The visual system functions as a very quick remote-sensing mechanism that alerts us to changes in the environment and enables us to identify threats and opportunities around us. The visual system is fairly well understood for normal adult populations in regard to the effects of light on both appearance (what things look like) and visual performance (how well visual information is processed). For example, there is a complete model of visual performance available for predicting the impact of background luminance (light level), target contrast, target size, and observer age from 18 to 65 years (Rea and Ouellette, 1991). Presumably, most school-age students should behave like 18-year-olds in regard to visual performance, but this has not been systematically studied. In general, given the characteristics of the visual response functions, it can probably be concluded that most lighting and task conditions are adequate for normal student visual performance. Going the next step, however, is more tenuous because there is no evidence that the quality or quantity of light directly affects student learning performance (Larson, 1965; Demos et al., 1967; Boyce et al., 2003).

Lighting for Visual Performance

The performance of any lighting design cannot be effectively evaluated solely on the basis of the source of illumination or the individual components needed to create the entire lighting system. Instead, lighting performance should be evaluated within the integrated system of enclosure design and controls, space geometry and finish, and fixture components in relation to the task requirements.

For a large majority of the people working in buildings, lighting for vision during the day is quite adequate, in part because people have very flexible visual systems and adjust their posture in response to the available lighting conditions. For example, the dimmer the light, the closer one holds the reading materials to maintain a constant ability to read. Experiments in the laboratory show that people will systematically adjust the eye-to-task geometry to maintain good task visibility, either by moving closer to the visual task or shifting posture to avoid reflected glare (Rea et al., 1985). A flexible visual system combined with a flexible body provides most people with the ability to adapt to less than ideal lighting environments.

A significant minority of the school-age population may not have properly corrected eyesight, however. Students without properly corrected eyesight may not be able to take full advantage of adaptive strategies to see learning materials in the classroom. In a large study using the 1996-1997 National Health Interview Survey, Kemper et al. (2004) determined that approximately 25 percent of school-age children in the United States have corrective lenses. They showed that the prevalence of corrective lenses is related to several population factors such as age (older children are more likely to wear corrective lenses), ethnicity (black and Hispanic children are less likely to wear corrective lenses), income (poorer children are less likely to wear corrective lenses), and gender (girls are more likely to wear corrective lenses than boys). Of particular note, insurance coverage appears to be a major factor in the prevalence of corrective lenses in school-age children. The actual percentage of corrective lenses probably underestimates the number of children who need them. Moreover, it is unknown whether students' corrective lenses actually have the proper refraction. Because lighting and task variables (e.g., particularly task target contrast and size) as well as proper refraction determine visual performance, it seems likely that at least some students are not able to adequately see learning materials in the classroom.

Within the context of the school environment, then, adequate lighting for the majority of the students may be insufficient for some fraction of school-age children. It could be hypothesized that for those students who do not have the proper refraction, daylight may offer a significant advantage by providing higher light levels and better geometries than would otherwise be present from electric lighting alone. However, the potential advantage of daylight in classrooms for improving visual performance of children with or without properly corrected eyesight has not been systematically studied.

The adult (teaching and administrative) population will also likely have problems with refractive errors. Normal aging involves a continuous loss of visual accommodative ability, known as presbyopia, from about 20 years of age to approximately 65 years (Weale, 1992). Until about age 45 the gradual loss in ability to focus on near objects is hardly noticed, but after this approximate age nearly everyone begins to adopt new strategies to see small targets. Instead of getting closer to an object to see it as they did when they were younger, people with presbyopia actually move the object further away from their eyes, or they place the object under a bright light, usually provided by a window or skylight. Eventually, everyone seeks optical aids, such as bifocals or reading glasses, to see normal print, but use of bright light from the right direction will continue to be a strategy employed by older people to see small targets throughout their lives.

Glare and Visual Performance

In regard to glare, there is much less certainty in predicting visual comfort, even in adults, than in predicting visual performance (Rea, 2000; Boyce, 2003). A clear distinction is made between glare that reduces visual performance (disability glare) and glare that does *not* (discomfort glare). Disability glare can be precisely predicted for a given individual and for the general population. As would be expected, disability glare becomes more problematic with age owing to changes in the optical media of the eye, particularly from scattering of light within the eye by the crystalline lens (Weale, 1963).

Windows are the largest sources of glare in a classroom. However, glare can be controlled by using fixed overhangs in conjunction with blinds or window treatments that can be manually operated. Methods to control light from skylights and clerestories are also needed because of ever-changing lighting geometries and light levels as the day progresses.

Formulas do exist for calculating discomfort glare, and these are often used to characterize the lighting layout for a space using commonly available lighting software. However, collective understanding of the mechanisms underlying discomfort glare is rather poor (Boyce, 2003). It appears that psychological phenomena contribute significantly to discomfort glare so that, for example, bright flashing lights in an office are highly uncomfortable, but the same lights can be highly desirable in a night club for dancing. Therefore, although disability glare is the same in both applications, discomfort glare is not. In this context, and given the strong psychological component to discomfort glare, predicting visual comfort in school-age children is an area that requires more research.

DAYLIGHTING AND STUDENT LEARNING

Several well-designed studies investigating the effect of daylighting on student performance were conducted by the Heschong-Mahone Group between 1999 and 2003. In the 1999 study, data were obtained from three elementary school districts located in Orange

County, California; Seattle, Washington; and Fort Collins, Colorado (Heschong-Mahone, 1999). The study looked for a correlation between the amount of daylight provided by each student's classroom environment and test scores. Test results for more than 21,000 students in these districts were analyzed. Demographic data sets, architectural plans, aerial photographs, the presence of skylights, maintenance records, and daylighting conditions for more than 2,000 classrooms were among the factors reviewed.

The study developed a regression model for approximately 150 independent variables (e.g., teacher salaries, grade level, attendance), including available daylight represented by five different levels, or "daylight codes." Although the regression analysis leads to a prediction that an increase in the value of the daylight code can increase scores in both math and English by more than 20 percent, a closer examination of the results shows that only 0.3 percent of the variance in the regression model is explained by daylight code (Boyce, 2004). This is a very small effect and one that cannot be justified as reliable. As noted below, these results could not be replicated in a subsequent study.

A reanalysis of the Capistrano and the Seattle school districts' data was undertaken in 2001 to look at additional variables that might have a confounding influence, including teacher assignments (Heschong-Mahone, 2001). In 2003 a third study was undertaken to see whether the original methodology and findings would hold when data came from a school district with a different climate and curriculum. The Fresno California school district was used. The preliminary statistical analyses replicated the structures of the models used in previous studies. In the Fresno study, the holistic variable called the Daylight Code "was not significant in predicting student performance. It had the least explanatory power of the variables considered, and the lowest significance level" (Heschong-Mahone, 2003, p. viii).

The authors proceeded with more detailed multilinear regression (statistical) analysis to see whether they could gain some insight into why the Daylight Code was not significant in Fresno as it had been in earlier studies. Among the authors' conclusions were that sources of glare negatively affect student learning; direct sun penetration into classrooms, especially through unshaded east or south facing windows, is associated with negative student performance, likely causing both glare and thermal discomfort; blinds or curtains allow teachers to control the intermittent sources of glare or visual distraction through their windows; when teachers do not have control of their windows, student performance is negatively affected (Heschong-Mahone, 2003, p. ix). They summarized that

> Characteristics describing windows were generally quite stable in their association with better or worse student performance. Variables describing a better view out of windows always entered the equations as positive and highly significant, while variables describing glare, sun penetration, and lack of visual control always entered the models as negative. (Heschong-Mahone, 2003, p. viii)

Because of the inconsistent results of this limited number of well-designed studies, there is insufficient evidence at this time to determine whether or not an association exists between daylighting and student learning.

LIGHTING AND THE CIRCADIAN SYSTEM

The circadian system involves biological rhythms that repeat at approximately 24-hour intervals. The behavior of all terrestrial species, including humans, is driven by an internal clock synchronized to the solar light-dark cycle. Indeed, light is the primary stimulus to the internal clock. The circadian system regulates not only overt daily patterns of behavior such as activity and rest, but also our bodies at the cellular level, regulating functions such as the cell cycle (Moore, 1997).

Current lighting technologies and lighting standards are designed exclusively for providing visual sensation. However, light affects the visual system very differently than it affects the circadian system. Relative to the visual system that underlies conventional photometry and all lighting standards, the circadian system needs a much higher light level on the retina for activation (McIntyre et al., 1989a,b); it has a peak spectral sensitivity to much shorter wavelengths (Brainard et al., 2001; Thapan et al., 2001); it has greater sensitivity to light in the inferior retina (viewing the sky) than in the superior retina (Glickman et al., 2003); it requires much longer exposures for activation (McIntyre et al., 1989a,b; Rea et al., 2002); and, most important, it is differentially sensitive to light depending on the time of day (Jewett et al., 1997).

There is a growing body of literature indicating that the effect of light on circadian regulation can affect productivity as well as health. Seasonal affective disorder (SAD), or the "winter blues," is recognized by the medical community as a psychiatric disorder. Apparently, seasonal reductions in the amount of daylight available in the winter at extreme northern (and southern) latitudes can induce depression (Rosen et al., 1990). Light treatment, typically provided with bright light from electric lighting systems, is recognized by the medical community as the preferred method of treating SAD (Rosenthal et al., 1985).

The incidence of SAD, or winter blues, in school-age children is poorly documented, although it has been reported that adults who experience SAD also experienced it as a child. It seems too that postpubescent young women are more likely to experience SAD (Rosenthal, 1998). Depending upon latitude, between 4 percent and 30 percent of the adult population, usually women, experience some symptoms of seasonal depression (Rosenthal, 1998), which in turn, might affect teachers. Less learning might be expected from those children who experience symptoms of seasonal depression, so lighting may play a very important role in the design of a green school at northern latitudes during the winter months. Systematic attempts to alleviate seasonal depression in children through lighting design have not been undertaken, but these early findings suggest a reconsideration of the role that light, particularly daylight, plays in the classroom.

Nearly half the population experiences some form of sleep disorder (National Sleep Foundation, 2005). Poor sleep directly affects a person's ability to perform tasks and learn new tasks (Jennings et al., 2003; Heuer et al., 2004). Light and dark have a dramatic impact on sleep quality (Turek and Zee, 1999; Reid and Zee, 2004). Adolescents in particular commonly go to sleep late (after midnight) and have difficulty getting up early (before 7:00 a.m.) to go to school (Carskadon et al., 1998). In extreme cases this difficulty in falling asleep early and getting up early is diagnosed as delayed sleep phase syndrome (DSPS). Many students with DSPS must get special training or even repeat grades because of poor attendance and poor performance. Light is a recognized treatment for this disorder, and a regular light-dark cycle may have broader implications for sleep quality in a larger group of children.

Recent research at the other end of the age spectrum shows that light treatment can consolidate sleep and increase sleep efficiency during the night in older people (Satlin et al., 1992; Fetveit et al., 2003; van Someren et al., 1997; Figueiro and Rea, 2005). A regimen of bright light at school during the day, together with dark nights at home, may increase student attendance and performance. Here again, however, there have been no systematic studies in school-age children.

DAYLIGHTING, VIEW, PERFORMANCE, AND HEALTH

Studies have been conducted using subjective ratings from adults providing evidence that people like views from windows (Markus, 1967; Jackson and Holmes, 1973; Ne'eman and Longmore, 1973; Collins, 1975; Ludlow, 1976; Cuttle, 1983; Heerwagen and Heerwagen, 1986; Leslie and Hartleb, 1990, 1991; Boubekri et al., 1991) and that real estate prices are higher for architectural spaces with a view from windows (Boyce et al., 2003). Kuller and Lindsten (1992) studied children's health and behavior in classrooms with and without windows for an entire academic year. At the end of the study, they concluded that work in classrooms without windows affected the basic pattern of the hormone cortisol, which is associated with stress. The authors concluded that windowless classrooms could have a negative effect on children's health and concentration. This finding is strictly suggestive, however, because no direct relationship between cortisol levels and student performance and health was established (Rusak et al., 1997).

FINDINGS AND RECOMMENDATIONS

Finding 4: In regard to lighting, performance, and health, the committee has found the following:

- Daylight is a special light source because it may provide a view (through a window), high light levels, and good color rendering, and it is ever-changing. Direct and reflected sunlight can create significant visual problems if windows, skylights, and clerestories allow in too much or too little light. However, such problems can be controlled with manual blinds and other types of window treatments.
- There is good evidence from studies of adult populations that the visual conditions in schools resulting from both electric lighting and daylighting are adequate for most children and adults.
- There is, however, concern that a significant percentage of students in classrooms do not have properly corrected eyesight, and thus, the general lighting conditions suitable for visual functioning by the average student may be inadequate for those students without properly corrected eyesight. It could be hypothesized that daylight may benefit these children by providing higher light levels and better geometries than would otherwise be present from electric lighting alone.

However, the potential advantages of daylight in classrooms for improving visual performance of children with or without properly corrected eyesight has not been systematically studied.

- Because of inconsistent results and the small number of well-designed studies, there is insufficient evidence at this time to determine whether or not an association exists between daylighting and student performance.
- A growing body of evidence suggests that lighting may play an important nonvisual role in human health and well-being through the circadian system. However, the effect of light on health through circadian regulation of sleep, depression, and cell cycle has not been directly studied in children.

Recommendation 2: To determine the potential and actual performance of a lighting system, the entire system should be assessed because the total performance cannot be effectively evaluated based solely on the source of illumination or on the individual components needed to create the entire lighting system.

Recommendation 3: For green schools in which the lighting strategy is to use daylight extensively, control systems that can be easily operated, such as manual blinds or other types of window treatments, should be specified in order to control excessive sunlight or glare.

5

Noise, Acoustics, Student Learning, and Teacher Health

Various studies show that noise exposure affects educational outcomes, and other research provides evidence of mechanisms to explain these effects of noise on learning. Speech intelligibility studies have found that students' ability to recognize speech sounds is decreased by even modest levels of ambient noise, and this effect is magnified for younger children. This problem may not be appreciated by adults, who are better able to recognize speech in the presence of noise.

Most learning in school classrooms involves speaking and listening as the primary communication modes: Students learn by listening to the teacher and to each other (Goodland, 1983). Excessive background noise or reverberation (i.e., many delayed reflections of the original sound) can interfere with speech perception and, consequently, can impair educational outcomes. Careful attention to acoustical design requirements is essential for creating an effective learning environment. Nonetheless, a 1995 report of the U.S. General Accounting Office estimated that approximately 22,000 U.S. schools attended by 11 million students had unsatisfactory acoustics for noise control: 28 percent of the schools in the survey reported unsatisfactory or very unsatisfactory environments related to acoustics for noise control (GAO, 1995a).

In 2002, the American National Standards Institute (ANSI) issued voluntary standard S12.60, "Acoustical Performance Criteria, Design Requirements, and Guidelines for Schools," which calls for a maximum ambient noise level of 35 dB(A) and includes recommendations for the required sound isolation between classrooms and adjacent spaces or the outdoors (ANSI, 2002). Many classrooms currently do not meet the recommendations of this standard, but at least one state, Connecticut, has already adopted the use of ANSI S12.60 for its schools.

People's ability to understand speech is influenced largely by the level of speech sounds relative to the level of ambient or background noise. Reverberant sound causes one word to smear into the next and can decrease the intelligibility of speech. Acoustical design involves designing to control sound to facilitate improvement in the perception of speech sounds. Controlling sound should focus primarily on reducing unwanted noise, and secondarily on controlling excessive reverberation. Good acoustical design can allow for more accurate verbal interaction and less repetition among teachers and students because spoken words are clearly understood, and as a consequence, it can facilitate learning. There is also evidence that good acoustical design may have a health benefit for teachers, by reducing the incidence of voice impairment.

Excessive noise can also interfere with learning by affecting memory (Hygge, 2003) and acting as a distraction that impairs a student's ability to pay attention. The ability to pay attention is most important when students are engaged in tasks that demand higher mental processes, such as learning new concepts or when teachers are verbally presenting new or complex information (Hartman, 1946). (See also Anderson, 2004, for a review of the effects of noise on children and classroom acoustics issues.)

Excessive background noise in a classroom can originate from outside the building (aircraft and traffic noise, lawnmowers and leaf blowing) or from within the building (heating, ventilation, air-conditioning, plumbing systems, noise from adjacent classrooms or hallways, gymnasiums or music rooms) or noise from the students themselves. However, it is important to note that the level of residual noise from the students is strongly related to the general level of ambient noise in the room. That is, student chatter will increase as the general level of ambient noise increases, an example of the Lombard effect (Junqua, 1996).

Speech perception studies have investigated how interference from noise and reverberation influences the perception of syllables, words, or sentences in classrooms. The importance of ambient noise levels is mostly related to speech-to-noise ratios. Kindergarten and first and second grades are the primary years in which children learn to break down written words into their phonetic components and acquire the ability to read. This requires careful listening to develop the ability to discriminate among minor differences in words such as pet, pit, pot, put, and pat (Anderson, 2004). Such differences can be lost in a noisy environment, and hence younger children require higher signal-to-noise ratios corresponding to quieter conditions.

The impacts of excessive noise vary according to the age of the students because

> the ability to focus on speech is a developmental skill that evolves with maturation of the brain and mastery of language. Because the auditory mechanism does not fully mature until age 13 to 15 years, young children . . . require better acoustical environments than do adult listeners to achieve equivalent word recognition scores. (Anderson, 2004, p. 119)

For that reason, a student's difficulty in understanding speech in noisy situations may not be recognized by teachers, building designers, or other adults. Said another way, adults cannot recognize the level of children's difficulty by using their own ability to perceive speech under the same adverse listening conditions. Elliott et al. (1979) found that the ability to recognize sentences in noisy environments improves systematically with age for children ages 7, 9, 11, 13, 15, and 17 years. This has recently been shown in extensive studies in actual classrooms (Bradley and Sato, 2004).

There are also studies suggesting that the negative effects of excessive reverberation are more acute for younger listeners (Nábělek and Robinson, 1982), but the requirements for children of various ages have not been determined. Although most standards (e.g., ANSI S12.60) recommend approximately a 0.6-s reverberation time, some studies have suggested that much shorter reverberation times would be better (Nábělek and Picket, 1974). However, some of these studies are flawed and their results cannot be relied upon. These experimental results are incomplete because they include only the negative effects of increased reverberation but not the positive benefits (i.e., increased speech levels). Further research is required to more precisely confirm optimum reverberation times for children of various ages.

NOISE AND STUDENT ACHIEVEMENT

Since the 1970s, a number of studies have been conducted that compare the reading skills of students in schools exposed to transportation noise with the reading skills of students in schools in quieter areas. A study in the early 1970s looked at the performance of children in a New York school that was parallel to the tracks of an elevated train. During a 3-year time period, a comparison of aggregate scores for students in grades two, four, and six was made between students on the noisy side and students on the nonnoisy side of the school. Students on the noisy side lagged behind in reading an average of 3 to 4 months compared with students on the quieter side. After the train tracks were treated to abate the noise, reading levels of children on what had been the noisier side of the building improved (Bronzaft and McCarthy, 1975; Bronzaft, 1981).

A 1982 study of students in New York schools under and not under flight paths matched the students for socioeconomic status, race, gender, hearing loss, mother's education level, and English as a second language (Green et al., 1982). The study found that high levels of environmental noise were inversely related to reading ability in elementary school children. A later study of students in New York matched students/schools for low socioeconomic status, student absentee rates, and teacher experience and then analyzed reading achievement test scores for grades two through six (Evans and Maxwell, 1997). The analysis found that a higher percentage of students in noisy schools were reading 1 to 2 years below their grade level.

A study of schools near Munich Airport looked at the cognitive effects on children when the airport was in operation and then after the airport was moved to a new location. The study found impaired reading comprehension in third and fourth grade children in schools located near the airport. Children from noisy communities had significantly more errors on a standardized reading test when compared with students from quieter communities. Further, reading comprehension deteriorated in children in schools near the new airport (Hygge et al., 1996).

A 1997 study comparing students from two schools near Heathrow Airport found a significant association between noise and reading comprehension that could not be accounted for by annoyance, social class, or other factors (Haines et al., 2001a,b).

In one of the most comprehensive and rigorous studies to date, Stansfeld et al. (2005) conducted a cross-national, cross-sectional study to assess the effect of exposure to aircraft and road traffic noise on cognitive performance (reading comprehension) and health in children. The study assessed 2,844 children ages 9 to 10 in 89 schools located in the United Kingdom, Spain, and the Netherlands in 2002. Schools in all three countries were selected on the basis of increasing levels of exposure to aircraft and traffic noise. The selected schools were matched by students' socioeconomic status, the primary language spoken at home, and other factors. External noise was measured, and reading comprehension was assessed using standardized and normalized tests routinely used in each country.

Tests were also conducted to measure students' recognition and recall (episodic memory), sustained attention, working memory, and prospective memory. Socioeconomic characteristics were assessed as potential confounding factors, and pilot studies were conducted to assess the feasibility, reliability, validity, and psychometric properties of the cognitive tests to be used. The pooled data gathered through the study were analyzed statistically using multilevel modeling, and the final results were adjusted for a number of factors including children's long-standing illness, parental support for schoolwork, and home ownership. The authors noted that the study's limitations were that it was cross-sectional, not longitudinal; was restricted to 9- and 10-year olds; did not focus on noise exposure in the students' homes; and used different noise assessment techniques in the three countries.

This study found that chronic exposure to aircraft noise "was associated with a significant impairment in reading comprehension. . . . [A] 5-decibel difference in aircraft noise was equivalent to a 2-month reading delay in the United Kingdom and a 1-month delay in the Netherlands" (Stansfeld et al., 2005, p. 1946). This outcome was consistent with findings from other studies on the effects of aircraft noise on reading comprehension. Because it was a cross-sectional study, the effect of long-term noise exposure to aircraft noise could not be measured. Socioeconomic status was not found to be a factor in the size of the effect, a finding that differs from findings of other studies. The study also found that aircraft noise was "not associated with impairment in working memory, prospective memory, or sustained attention" (Stansfeld et al., 2005, p. 1946).

Stansfeld et al. (2005) also looked at the effect of traffic noise on the children. The authors noted linear exposure-effect associations between exposure to road traffic noise and increased functioning of episodic memory, in regard to information and conceptual recall (Stansfeld et al., 2005, p. 1947).

NOISE AND TEACHERS' HEALTH

Teachers who work in noisy classrooms must constantly raise their voices to be heard over various other sounds. Over time, this can lead to vocal fatigue and other voice problems. One study published in 1993 found that four out of five teachers who participated in the study indicated some problems with vocal fatigue (Gotaas and Starr, 1993). A 1995 study of populations in the U.S. workforce that rely on voice as a primary tool of their trade found that teachers constitute more than 20 percent of the voice-clinic load or five times the number expected by their prevalence in this segment of the workforce (Titze et al., 1996).

FINDINGS AND RECOMMENDATION

Finding 5: In regard to noise, acoustics, student learning, and teacher health, the committee has found the following:

- Sufficient evidence exists to conclude that there is an association between decreased noise levels in schools and improvement in student achievement.
- Although there is strong evidence that reduced noise levels are most important for younger children because they are still developing speech discrimination, additional research is required to more precisely define possible needs for control of reverberant sound for younger children.
- Some available evidence indicates that teacher health, in regard to voice impairment, may be adversely affected by noisier environments, although the magnitude of the effect cannot currently be estimated as a function of exposure to noise.

Recommendation 4: To facilitate student learning, guidelines for green schools should include requirements to meet American National Standards Institute (ANSI) Standard S12.60, "Acoustical Performance Criteria, Design Requirements, and Guidelines for Schools."

6

Building Condition and Student Achievement

For more than two decades, professional organizations and governmental agencies have been reporting on the condition of the nation's schools (AASA, 1983; Council of Great City Schools, 1987; Educational Writers' Association, 1989; GAO, 1995a,b; NEA, 2000).[7] These reports have consistently found that a substantial portion of the school-age population was being educated in substandard buildings. And schools with the highest concentrations of students from low-income households were more likely to be in substandard condition.

In *School Facilities: Condition of America's Schools*, the U.S. General Accounting Office estimated that approximately 14 million students (30 percent of all students) attended schools that needed extensive repairs or replacement (one-third of the school inventory) (GAO, 1995a). Approximately 28 million students attended schools that needed extensive repairs on one or more major building systems. The building components or features most often identified as needing attention in substandard schools were proper thermal control (temperature and humidity), ventilation, plumbing, roofs, exterior walls, finishes, windows, doors, electrical power, electrical lighting, life safety (fire suppression), and interior finishes and trims. The cost to make necessary repairs was estimated at more than $100 billion (1995 dollars). The state of Massachusetts was included in this survey, and the condition of the school buildings in that state reflected the condition of schools nationwide.

A second GAO report, *School Facilities: America's Schools Not Designed or Equipped for 21st Century,* found that approximately 40 percent of the schools surveyed could not meet the functional requirements of laboratory science or large-group instruction (GAO, 1995b). About two-thirds of the schools reported that they could not support educational reform measures such as a private space for counseling and testing, parental support activities, social/health care, day care, and before- and after-school care.

In 2000 the U.S. National Center for Educational Statistics reported that at least 29 percent of the nation's schools had problems with heating, ventilation, and air-conditioning; 25 percent had plumbing problems; 24 percent reported problems with exterior walls, finishes, windows, and doors; and about 20 percent had less than adequate conditions for life safety, roofs, and electrical power. About 11 million students attended school in the school districts reporting buildings with less than adequate condition. Of these students, approximately 3.5 million students attended schools in which the condition was rated as poor, replacement was needed, or significant substandard performance was apparent (NCES, 2000).

The National Education Association (NEA) has estimated it would cost $322 billion to repair, modernize, retrofit for new technology, and make major improvements to existing school buildings (NEA, 2000). This figure also included new construction and additions to

---

[7] Note: The studies referred to in this chapter use building condition as a qualitative and quantitative measure of a variety of systems and components. In some cases, these conditions included problems related to moisture in buildings, acoustics, lighting, and so forth. Thus, building condition is not necessarily separate from the issues discussed in Chapters 2 through 5.

existing buildings, which explains the disparity with earlier estimates. For the state of Massachusetts, the cost to improve all existing buildings is estimated to range from $8.9 billion to $9.9 billion.

Implicit in these reports is the underlying assumption that school condition and functionality can influence student learning, either positively or negatively. Although most school buildings start out meeting current codes, standards, and functional design, over time physical conditions deteriorate if building components and systems are not properly operated and maintained or repaired in a timely manner.

SCHOOL BUILDING CONDITION AND STUDENT ACHIEVEMENT

The committee identified seven studies that investigated the relationship between the condition of school buildings and at least two student variables. The one consistent variable was student achievement as measured by some form of standardized or normed test or examination administered to all students in the schools. Four of the seven studies focused on high school students, one focused on third and fifth graders, and two included students at elementary, middle, and high school levels. A description of each of the studies, the methodology used, the reported findings, and the committee's conclusions follow.

Edwards (1992) investigated the relationship between parental involvement, school building condition, and student achievement in the schools of Washington, D.C. She hypothesized that the condition of public school buildings is affected by parental involvement and that the condition of the school building further affects student achievement. She analyzed these relationships by evaluating the condition of school buildings, determining the extent of parental involvement and the amount of funds parents raised for the local school, and compared the results with student achievement scores, as measured using average test scores on the Comprehensive Test of Basic Skills (CTBS).

Edwards found that building condition did have an effect on student achievement scores. The analysis indicated that as a school moves up from one condition category to another (e.g., from poor to fair), the achievement scores can be expected to increase by 5 percent. If the school moves up two categories, such as from poor to excellent, the average achievement scores can be expected to increase by 11 percent.

In a similar study, Cash (1993) investigated the relationship between certain school building conditions, student achievement, and student behavior in rural high schools in Virginia. Basically, the same hypothesis that Edwards employed was used in conducting this study. The condition of the building in this study, however, was the independent variable, and student achievement and behavior served as dependent variables.

The condition of the school building was determined through evaluation by local school system personnel. Cash developed a building evaluation instrument, the Commonwealth Assessment of Physical Environment (CAPE), to be used by local school personnel to determine the classification of the building. The CAPE was derived from previous studies that showed a positive relationship between a particular building condition and student achievement and behavior, including air-conditioning, classroom illumination, temperature control, classroom color, graffiti, science equipment and utilities, paint schedules, roof adequacy, classroom windows, floor type, building age, supporting facilities, condition of school grounds, and furniture condition. The presence or absence of these factors determined the overall condition of the building: substandard, standard, and above standard.

Student achievement was measured by use of scaled scores of students taking the Test of Academic Proficiency (TAP), which was administered to all 11th grade students in Virginia. The ratio of students receiving free and reduced lunches was used to control for socioeconomic status of the school attendance area, and the Virginia Composite Index was used as a measure of local fiscal capacity, to control for the wealth of the school jurisdiction.

The data analysis was done by comparing achievement score means of building condition ratings using analysis of covariance to adjust the means. The percentage of students who did not qualify for free or reduced lunch was the covariant. The adjusted mean scale scores in achievement and the behavior ratios for each building were compared across the three levels of building condition and between the three levels of overall, cosmetic, and structural categories. Cash found significant differences between the achievement scores of students in poor buildings and those in above-standard buildings when the overall condition of the building was used as a measure. She also found a larger number of differences in scores of students when the cosmetic features of a building were used as a measure of comparison. She observed that apparently students were more aware of the cosmetic than the structural condition of a building. The difference between test scores of students in poor and above-standard buildings ranged from 2 to 5 percentile points, depending on the subtest.

Earthman et al. (1996) used a similar methodology to conduct a study in North Dakota that included all 199 high school buildings in the state. North Dakota was selected for the study because traditionally students as a whole score among the highest in the nation on the Scholastic Aptitude Test. North Dakota students also scored third highest in the International Comparison of 8th Grade Math scores in 1992, behind only Asia and Japan (Leadership News, 1994). The state has a relatively homogeneous, mostly rural population.

Although the differences in the composite score were exactly the same as for the Cash study, there are some notable differences. The CTBS has additional subtests that the TAP does not have, such as reading, vocabulary, mathematics concepts, and spelling. The differences in reading, vocabulary, and spelling are rather high, considering the differences in other subtests. The North Dakota study does support the findings of both the Edwards and the Cash studies. Both of these researchers found at least a 5 percent difference in composite achievement scores in their population. The North Dakota study found a similar difference in percentile rankings in student achievement scores.

Hines (1996) used the same methodology and data-gathering instrument as Cash to study large urban high schools in Virginia. His results in comparing building condition and student achievement were basically the same. The range of differences between substandard and above-standard buildings, however, was greater than what was found in the study of rural high schools and in the North Dakota high schools study. In the Hines study, differences in test scores for students in above-standard schools ranged from 9 points higher for writing and science, to 15 points higher for reading, and 17 points higher for mathematics compared with the test scores of students in substandard buildings. This compares favorably with the results Edwards obtained in her comparison between the worst and best school buildings. Edwards stated that the difference in mean achievement scores for her study population was as much as 10.9 percent between school buildings in the substandard and above-standard categories (p. 24).

Lanham (1999) completed a study of the relationship between classroom conditions and student achievement in the elementary schools of Virginia that housed both third- and fifth-grade students. The researcher used the same general approach to investigating this relationship as Cash (1993) did on the high school level. From a total of 989 elementary schools, a random sample of 299 schools was drawn. Responses were received from 197 schools, representing a 66 participation rate. Lanham concluded that although certain school building and cosmetic components and features have a part in explaining the variance in student achievement scores, the socioeconomic status of the student as represented by participation in the free and reduced lunch program accounts for the most variance.

Schneider (2002) investigated the relationship between the condition of school buildings and student achievement scores in two large urban school districts, Washington, D.C., and Chicago, Illinois. In testing for the relationship between student achievement and building condition, the researcher used the results of the reading and or math scores on the Stanford Achievement Test in Washington, D.C., and the Iowa Test of Basic Skills in Chicago.

In Washington the difference in achievement scores was reported as the percent of students performing above the basic level of achievement for the grade. In Chicago the difference was reported as the percent of students performing at grade level. After controlling for factors such as poverty, ethnicity, and school size, the researcher was able to report a difference in both cities of between 3 to 4 percentage points in performance between students in poor buildings and those in good buildings. In other words, the students in schools with good conditions were performing from 3 to 4 percentage points better than students in buildings with poor conditions. In Washington, the difference was 3 percent in both reading and math between students in good and poor buildings. In Chicago, the difference was 3 percent for reading and 4 percent for math scores. These differences are well within the range of differences reported by other researchers.

Lewis (2000) conducted a study in the Milwaukee public schools comparing building condition with student achievement scores. The school system had approximately 139 elementary, middle, and high school buildings. All buildings were evaluated for both condition and adequacy. The Wisconsin Student Assessment System (WSAS) was used to measure student achievement. The WSAS consisted of three sets of standardized tests administered in the fourth, eighth, and tenth grades. Students were assessed in reading, mathematics, language arts and writing, science, and social studies. Scores on these examinations were reported as a percentage of students in each school building who were achieving at or above the level defined as proficient in the subject. These percentages were converted to standardized scores with a mean of 100 for analysis purposes. WSAS scores for 1996, 1997, and 1998 were used. Data were also gathered on student demographics, race, attendance, truancy, suspensions, mobility, and participation in school lunch programs. Multiple regression analyses were conducted. The overall hypothesis of the study was that as the condition of the school building increased, student test scores would also increase.

The study demonstrated several significant relationships, yet the findings were not consistent. Based on these results, Lewis (2000) concluded that the "significant relationships for facility measurements typically explain about 10 to 15 percent of the differences in scores across schools when the influences of the other variables were statistically controlled" (p. 11). When comparing student demographic indicators such as mobility rates, eligibility for free/reduced lunches, attendance, and suspensions, only 9 estimates out of 48 were found to be significant. Thus those indicators that were significant explained between 8 and 28 percent of the difference between test scores when other variables were controlled.

SCHOOL BUILDING FUNCTIONALITY AND STUDENT ACHIEVEMENT

Eleven studies were identified that investigated the relationship between school building functionality and student achievement. In each study, the age of the school building was used as a surrogate for functionality. The age of a building may not in and of itself be a direct negative factor in student achievement, but what qualities the building does not have might provide a direct relationship to student achievement. Building age might also serve as a surrogate for a number of specific variables such as condition of the building, thermal control, proper lighting, acoustical control, support facilities, condition of laboratories, aesthetic condition, among others.

Under the variable of school building age, McGuffey (1982) reviewed seven studies (Thomas, 1962; Burkhead et al., 1967; Michelson, 1970; Guthrie et al., 1971; McGuffey and Brown, 1978, Plumley, 1978; and Chan, 1979). In all cases, increasing building age was significant as a factor detrimental to student achievement and behavior; i.e., as building age increased, student achievement decreased.

McGuffey and Brown (1978) studied 188 school districts in Georgia to explore the relationship between building age and student achievement. They used the scores on the Iowa Test of Basic Skills for the fourth and eighth grade students and the Test of Academic Progress for eleventh grade students. In comparing student test scores with the age of the building, the statistical analyses indicated that building age could account for 0.5 percent to 2.6 percent of the variance among fourth grade students, 0 percent to 2.6 percent of the variance among eighth grade students, and 1.4 percent to 3.3 percent of the variance among eleventh graders.

In addition to the studies above, Garrett (1981), Chan (1982), Bowers and Burkett (1989), and Phillips (1997) conducted similar studies using age of the building as an independent variable and student achievement test scores as dependent variables. Their findings substantiated those of previous studies.

Students in the new school building significantly outperformed the students in the older building in reading, listening, language, and arithmetic. Further, faculty in the new building reported fewer disciplinary incidents and health problems than did faculty in the old building. Attendance likewise was better for students in the new building than for students in the old school. Researchers conducting these studies concluded that a relationship did exist between the physical environment and student achievement, health, attendance, and behavior.

In all of the studies cited above, the range of difference between the test scores of students in substandard and standard school buildings was between 1 and 17 percentile points. In almost all cases there was a positive difference for students in the better buildings. These findings are of particular importance because of the large number of school buildings across the United States that are in substandard condition.

All of these studies raise the important question, If students are housed in poor buildings for a number of years, will the negative effect on achievement be multiplied the longer a student is in these buildings? The research cited here is simply a snapshot of conditions and relationships at one period of time, not over successive periods of time. There is a reasonable basis to believe, however, that the harmful effect of poor school buildings on student test scores may be cumulative and may continue to worsen the longer the student is in school.

The condition of existing buildings results from the amount of attention to maintenance that the buildings have had over the years. Assuming the original building is constructed of quality materials with good workmanship applied, the normal life of a well-built school is at least 30 years. During this period of time proper maintenance is required to keep the building in as good a condition as when it was initially constructed. Lack of attention to maintaining the building in good condition results in deterioration of the structure and all of its systems, and the life expectancy of the building is reduced.

LIMITATIONS OF THE CURRENT STUDIES

One factor that can have an influence on the results of a research study devoted to the investigation of the relationship between school building condition and student achievement is the method used to evaluate the condition of a building. There is no statistical evidence to indicate that using one kind of building assessment method or instrument is better than using another. Nevertheless, the studies that have used instruments designed to gauge maintenance and its effects have not been as successful in finding relationships as those studies that have used instruments designed to study the performance of occupants. This leads one to believe that a focus on assessment of a building does limit the results of some studies.

The studies that used the age of a building or the condition of a school building as an independent variable in comparing student achievement test scores have the same limitations as cited above. As in almost all studies using student achievement scores, there is the limitation of not being able to control all of the variables associated with student learning Variables such as the quality of the teaching staff, the curriculum, the viability of the student test measures, and, most important, the background of the student are all virtually impossible to completely control For this reason the evidence found in these studies concerning the relationship between school building age and student achievement must be considered as a suggestive association.

FINDING AND RECOMMENDATION

Finding 6: In regard to building condition and student achievement, the committee found the following:

- The body of available research is suggestive of an association between the condition of a school building and student achievement. All of the studies analyzed by the committee found that student test scores improved as the physical condition of school buildings improved. The degree of improvement of students' test scores varied across the studies, but in all cases students in buildings in better condition scored higher than students in buildings in poor condition.

Recommendation 5: Guidelines for green schools should place significant emphasis on operations and maintenance practices if potential health and productivity benefits are to be achieved and maintained over the lifetime of a building.

References

AASA (American Association of School Administrators). 1983. The Maintenance Gap: Deferred Repair and Renovation in the Nation's Elementary and Secondary Schools. Arlington, VA: AASA.

Anderson, K. 2004. The problem of classroom acoustics: The typical classroom soundscape is a barrier to learning. Semin. Hearing 25:117-129.

ANSI (American National Standards Institute). 2002. Standard S12.60. Acoustical Performance Criteria, Design Requirements and Guidelines for Schools. Washington, DC: ANSI.

ANSI (American National Standards Institute). 2004. Building Commissioning. Washington, DC: ANSI.

ANSI/ASHRAE. 2004. Standard 55-2004. Thermal Environmental Conditions for Human Occupancy. Washington, DC: ANSI.

ASHRAE (American Society of Heating, Refrigeration, and Air Conditioning Engineers). 2004. Standard 62.1. Ventilation for Acceptable Indoor Air Quality. Washington, DC: ASHRAE.

Belanger, K., Beckett, W., Triche, E., Bracken, M.B., Holford, T., Ren, P., McSharry, J.E., Gold, D.R., Platts-Mills, T.A., and Leaderer, B.P. 2003. Symptoms of wheeze and persistent cough in the first year of life: Associations with indoor allergens, air contaminants and maternal history of asthma. Am. J. Epidemiol. 158:195-202.

Bloom, B., and Tonthat, L. 2002. Summary health statistics for U.S. children: National health interview survey, 1997. Vital Health Stat. Series 10, 203:1-46.

Boubekri, M., Hull, R.B., and Boyer, L.L. 1991. Impact of window size and sunlight penetration on office workers' mood and satisfaction: A novel way of assessing sunlight. Environment and Behavior 23(4):474-493.

Bowers, J.H., and Burkett, C.W. 1989. Effects of physical and school environment on students and faculty. Educational Facility Planner 27(1):28-29.

Boyce, P.R. 2003. Human Factors in Lighting, 2nd Edition. London and New York: Taylor and Francis.

Boyce, P.R. 2004. Reviews of Technical Reports on Daylight and Productivity. Troy, NY: Lighting Research Center. Available at www.daylightdividends.org.

Boyce, P.R., Hunter, C., and Howlett, O. 2003. The benefits of daylight through windows. Report submitted to Capturing the Daylight Dividends Program. Troy, NY: Lighting Research Center. Available at www.daylightdividends.org.

Bradley, J.S., and Sato, H. 2004. Speech intelligibility test results for grades 1, 3 and 6. Children in Real Classrooms. Paper Tu4B1.2. Proceedings of the 18th International Congress on Acoustics. Kyoto, Japan.

Brainard, G.C., Hanifin, J.P., Greeson, J.M., Byrne, B., Glickman, G., Gerner, E., and Rollag, M.D. 2001. Action spectrum for melatonin regulation in humans: Evidence for a novel circadian photoreceptor. J. Neurosci. 21(16):6405-6412.

Bronzaft, A.L. 1981. The effect of a noise abatement program on reading ability. J. Environ. Psychol. 1:215-222.

Bronzaft, A.L., and McCarthy, D.P. 1975. The effect of elevated train noise on reading ability. J. Environ. Behav. 7:517-528.

Burkhead, J., Fox, T., and Holland, J.W. 1967. Input and Output in Large-City High Schools. Syracuse, NY: Syracuse University Press.

Carskadon, M.A., Wolfson, A.R., Acebo, C., Tzischinsky, O., and Seifer, R. 1998. Adolescent sleep patterns, circadian timing, and sleepiness at a transition to early school days. Sleep 21(8):871-881.

Cash, C.S. 1993. Building condition and student achievement and behavior. Unpublished doctoral dissertation. Blacksburg, VA: Virginia Polytechnic Institute and State University.

CDC (Centers for Disease Control and Prevention). 2004. Asthma Prevalence, Health Care Use and Mortality, 2002. Hyattsville, MD: U.S. Department of Health and Human Services.

Chan, T.C. 1979. The impact of school building age on the achievement of eighth-grade pupils from the public schools in the state of Georgia. Unpublished doctoral dissertation. Athens, GA: University of Georgia.

Chan, T.C. 1982. A comparative study of pupil attitudes toward new and old school buildings. Greenville, SC: Greenville County School District. ERIC Document Reproduction Service No. ED 222 981.

CHPS (Collaborative for High Performance Schools). 2004. Best Practices Manual. Volumes 1-4. Available at www.chps.net.

CHPS. 2005. Web site at www.chps.net. Accessed October 31, 2005.

Collins, B.L. 1975. Windows and People: A Literature Survey: Psychological Reaction to Environments with and Without Windows. National Bureau of Standards Building Science Series 70. Washington, DC: U.S. Department of Commerce.

Council of Great City Schools. 1987. Report on Deferred Maintenance to the Council of the Great City Schools. Washington, DC: Council of Great City Schools.

Cox-Ganser, J.M., White, S.K, Jones, R., Hilsbos, K., Storey, E., Enright, P.L., Rao, C.Y., and Kreiss, K. 2005. Respiratory morbidity in office workers in a water damaged building. Environ. Health Perspect. 113:485-490.

Cuttle, K. 1983. People and windows in workplaces. Pp. 203-212 in Proceedings of the People and Physical Environment Research Conference. Wellington, New Zealand.

Daisey, J.M., Angell, W.J., and Apte, M.G. 2003. Indoor air quality, ventilation, and health symptoms in schools: An analysis of existing information. Indoor Air 13:53-64.

Darling-Hammond, L. 1999. Teacher Quality and Student Achievement: A Review of State Policy Evidence. Seattle, WA: University of Washington.

Deal, B.M., Rose, W., and Riley, S.E. 1998. Commissioning for humidified buildings. USACERL Technical Report 99/03. Champaign, IL: U.S. Army Corps of Engineers Construction Engineering Research Laboratories.

Demos, G.D., Davis, S., and Zuwaylif, F.F. 1967. Controlled physical environments. Building Research 4:60-62.

Earthman, G.I., Cash, C.S., and Van Berkum, D. 1996. Student achievement and behavior and school building condition. J. School Business Management 8(3):26-37.

Educational Writers Association. 1989. Wolves at the Schoolhouse Door: An Investigation of the Conditions of Public School Buildings. Washington, DC: Educational Writers Association.

Edwards, M.M. 1992. Building conditions, parental involvement and student achievement in the D.C. public school system. Unpublished master's thesis. Washington, DC: Georgetown University.

Elliott, L., Connors, S., Kille, E., Levin, S., Ball, K., and Katz, D. 1979. Children's understanding of monosyllabic nouns in quiet and in noise. J. Acoust. Soc. Am. 66:12-21.

Evans, G.W., and Maxwell, L. 1997. Chronic noise exposure and reading deficits. J. Environ. Behav. 29(5):638-656.

Fang, L., Clausen, G., and Fanger, P.O. 1998. Impact of temperature and humidity on the perception of indoor air quality. Indoor Air 8:80-90.

Fanger, P.O. 2000. Indoor air quality in the 21st century: The search for excellence. Indoor Air 10:68-73.

Federspiel, C.C., Fisk, W.J., Price, P.N., Liu, G., Faulkner, D., Dibartolomeo, D.L., Sullivan, D.P., and Lahiff, M. 2004. Worker performance and ventilation in a call center: Analyses of work performance data for registered nurses. Indoor Air 14(Suppl 8):41-50.

Fetveit, A., Skjerve, A., and Bjorvatn, B. 2003. Bright light treatment improves sleep in institutionalized elderly—An open trial. Int. J. Geriatr. Psychiatry 18(6):520-526.

FFC (Federal Facilities Council). 2005. Implementing Health-Protective Features and Practices in Buildings. Washington, DC: The National Academies Press.

Figueiro, M.G., and Rea, M.S. 2005. LEDs: Improving the sleep quality of older adults. Proceedings of the CIE Midterm Meeting and International Lighting Congress. Leon, Spain, May 18-21.

GAO (General Accounting Office). 1995a. School Facilities: Condition of America's Schools. GAO/HEHS-95-61.Washington, DC: GAO.

GAO. 1995b. School Facilities: America's Schools Not Designed or Equipped for 21st Century. GAO/HEHS-955-95. Washington, DC: GAO.

Garrett, D.M. 1981. The impact of school building age on the academic achievement of high school pupils in the state of Georgia. Unpublished doctoral dissertation. Athens, GA: University of Georgia.

Glickman, G., Hanifin, J.P., Rollag, M.D., Wang, J., Cooper, H., and Brainard, G.C. 2003. Inferior retinal light exposure is more effective than superior retinal exposure in suppressing melatonin in humans. J. Biol. Rhythms 18(1):71-79.

Goodland, J. 1983. A Place Called School. Prospects for the Future. New York: McGraw-Hill.

Gotaas, C., and Starr, C.C. 1993. Vocal fatigue among teachers. Folia Phoniatr. (Basel) 45:120-129.

Green, K.B., Pasternack, B.S., and Shore, R.E. 1982. Effects of aircraft noise on reading ability of school-age children. Arch. Environ. Health 37:24-31.

Guthrie, J.W., Kleindorfer, G.B., Levin, H.M., and Stout, R.T. 1971. Schools and Inequity. Cambridge, MA: MIT Press.

Haines, M.M., Stansfeld, S.A., and Brentnall, S. 2001a. The West London School Study: The effects of chronic aircraft noise exposure on child health. Psychol. Med. 3:1385-1396.

Haines, M.M., Stansfeld, S.A., Job, R., Berglund, B., and Hea, J. 2001b. Chronic noise exposure, stress responses, mental health and cognitive performance in schools. Psychol. Med. 31:265-277.

Hartman, G. 1946. The effects of noise on children. J. Educ. Psychol. 37:149-161.

Heerwagen, J., and Heerwagen, D. 1986. Lighting and psychological comfort. Lighting Design and Application 6:47-51.

Heschong-Mahone Group. 1999. Daylighting in Schools: An Investigation into the Relationship Between Daylighting and Human Performance. Fair Oaks, CA: Heschong-Mahone Group.

Heschong-Mahone Group. 2001. Daylighting in Schools: Reanalysis Report. Technical Report P500-03-082-A-3. Sacramento, CA: California Energy Commission.

Heschong-Mahone Group. 2003. Windows and Classrooms: A Study of Student Performance and the Indoor Environment. P500-03-082-A-7. Fair Oaks, CA: Heschong-Mahone Group.

Heuer, H., Kleinsorge, T., Klein, W., and Kohlisch, O. 2004. Total sleep deprivation increases the costs of shifting between simple cognitive tasks. Acta Psychol. (Amst.) 117(1):29-64.

Hines, E.C. 1996. Building condition and student achievement and behavior. Unpublished doctoral dissertation. Blacksburg, VA: Virginia Polytechnic Institute and State University.

Hygge, S. 2003. Classroom experiments on the effects of different noise sources and sound levels on long-term recall and recognition in children. Appl. Cognit. Psychol. 17:895-914.

Hygge, S., Evans, G.W., and Bullinger, M. 1996. The Munich Airport noise study: Cognitive effects on children from before to after the change of airports. Proceedings of Internoise '96 5:2189-2194. Liverpool.

IOM (Institute of Medicine). 1991. Adverse Effects of Pertussis and Rubella Vaccines. Washington, DC: National Academy Press.

IOM. 1993. Adverse Events Associated with Childhood Vaccines: Evidence Bearing on Causality. Stratton, K.R., Howe, C.J., and Johnston, R.B., eds. Washington, DC: National Academy Press.

IOM. 1994. Veterans and Agent Orange: Health Effects of Herbicides Used in Vietnam. Washington, DC: National Academy Press.

IOM. 1996. Veterans and Agent Orange. Update 1996. Washington, DC: National Academy Press.

IOM. 1999. Veterans and Agent Orange. Update 1998. Washington, DC: National Academy Press.

IOM. 2000. Clearing the Air: Asthma and Indoor Air Exposures. Washington, DC: National Academy Press.

IOM. 2003. Veterans and Agent Orange. Update 2002. Washington, DC: The National Academies Press.

IOM. 2004. Damp Indoor Spaces and Health. Washington, DC: The National Academies Press.

Jaakola, M.S., Nordman, H., Piipari, R., Uitti, J., Laitinen, J., and Karjalainen, A. 2002. Indoor dampness and molds and development of adult-onset asthma: A population-based incident study. Environ. Health Perspect. 110:543-547.

Jackson, G.J., and Holmes, J.G. 1973. Let's keep it simple—What we want from daylight. Light and Lighting 12:80-82.

Jennings, J.R., Monk, T.H., and van der Molen, M.W. 2003. Sleep deprivation influences some but not all processes of supervisory attention. Psychol. Sci. 14(5):473-479.

Jewett, M., Rimmer, D.W., Duffy, J.F., Klerman, E.B., Kronauer, R., and Czeisler, C.A. 1997. Human circadian pacemaker is sensitive to light throughout subjective day without evidence of transients. Am. J. Physiol. 273:R1800-R1809.

Junqua, J.C. 1996. The influence of acoustics on speech production: A noise-induced stress phenomenon known as the Lombard reflex. Speech Commun. 20:13-22.

Kemper, A.R., Bruckman, D., and Freed, G.L. 2004. Prevalence and distribution of corrective lenses among school-age children. Optom. Vis. Sci. 81(1):7-10.

Kuller, R., and Lindsten, C. 1992. Health and behavior of children in classrooms with and without windows. J. Environ. Psychol. 12:305-317.

Lanham III, J.W. 1999. Relating building and classroom conditions to student achievement in Virginia's elementary schools. Unpublished doctoral dissertation. Blacksburg, VA: Virginia Polytechnic Institute and State University.

Larson, C.T. 1965. The effect of windowless classrooms on elementary school children. Architectural Research Laboratory, Department of Architecture, University of Michigan, Ann Arbor.

Leadership News. 1994. Performance-Based Funds to Finance Educational Reforms. August 15, p. 4.

Leslie, R., and Hartleb, S. 1990. Windows, variability, and human response. Proceedings of the International Daylighting Conference. Moscow.

Leslie, R., and Hartleb, S. 1991. Some effects of the sequential experience of windows on human response. J. Illuminating Engineering Society, Winter, pp. 91-99.

Lewis, M.G. 2000. Facility Condition and Student Test Performance in the Milwaukee Public Schools. ED 459 593. Scottsdale, AZ: Council of Educational Facility Planners, International.

Lstiburek, J., and Carmody, J. 1994. The Moisture Control Handbook: Principles and Practices for Residential and Small Commercial Buildings. New York: John Wiley & Sons.

Ludlow, A.M. 1976. The functions of windows in buildings. Lighting Research and Technology 6(2):57-68.

Maier, W.C., Arrighi, H.M., Murray, B., Llewellyn, and Redding, G.C. 1997. Indoor risk factors for asthma and wheezing among school children. Environ. Health Perspect. 105:208-214.

Maniccia, D., Rutledge, B., Rea, M., and Narendran, N. 1998. A field study of lighting controls. Lighting Research Center, Rensselaer Polytechnic Institute, Troy, NY.

Mannino, D., Homa, D., Akinbami, L., Moorman, J., Gwynn, C., and Redd, S. Centers for Disease Control and Prevention. Surveillance for asthma prevalence-United States 1980-1999.

Markus, T.A. 1965. The function of windows: A reappraisal. Building Science 2:97-121.

McGuffey, C.W. 1982. *Facilities*. Chapter 10. Pp. 237-288 in W. Herbert, ed., Improving Educational Standards and Productivity. Berkeley, CA: McCutchan Publishing Corp.

McGuffey, C.W., and Brown, C.L. 1978. The impact of school building age on school achievement in Georgia. CEFP Journal 16:6-9.

McIntyre, I.M., Norman, T.R., Burrows, G.D., and Armstrong, S.M. 1989a. Human melatonin suppression by light is intensity dependent. J. Pineal Res. 6(2):149-156.

McIntyre, I.M., Norman, T.R., Burrows, G.D., and Armstrong, S.M. 1989b. Quantal melatonin suppression by exposure to low intensity light in man. Life Sci. 45(4):327-332.

Mendell, M.J., and Heath, G.A. 2004. Do indoor pollutants and thermal conditions in schools influence student performance? A critical review of the literature. Indoor Air 15:27-52.

Michelson, S. 1970. The Association of Teacher Resourcefulness with Children's Characteristics. Do Teachers Make a Difference? A Report on Recent Research on Pupil

Achievement. U.S. Office of Education Report OE-58042. Washington, DC: U.S. Government Printing Office.

Milton, K., Glenross, P., and Walters, M. 2000. Risk of sick leave associated with outdoor air supply rate, humidification, and occupant complaint. Int. J. Indoor Air Quality and Climate 10:211-221.

Moore, R.Y. 1997. Circadian rhythms: Basic neurobiology and clinical applications. Annu. Rev. Med. 48:253-266.

Nábělek, A.K., and Pickett, J.M. 1974. Reception of consonants in a classroom as affected by monaural and binaural listening, noise, reverberation, and hearing aids. J. Acoust. Soc. Am. 56(2):628-639.

Nábělek, A.K., and Robinson, P.K. 1982. Monaural and binaural speech perception in reverberation for listeners of various ages. J. Acoust. Soc. Am. 71(5):1242-1248.

National Sleep Foundation. 2005. Sleep in America Poll. Available at http://www.sleepfoundation.org/_content/hottopics/2005_summary_of_findings.pdf. Accessed September 20, 2005.

NCES (National Center for Education Statistics). 2000. Condition of America's Public School Facilities: 1999. NCES2000-032. Washington, DC: U.S. Department of Education.

NEA (National Education Association). 2000. Modernizing Our Schools: What Will It Cost? Washington, DC: NEA.

Ne'eman, E., and Longmore, J. 1973. Physical aspects of windows: Integration of daylight with artificial light. Proceedings of CIE Conference on Windows and Their Function in Architectural Design. Istanbul.

NORDAMP (Nordic Interdisciplinary Review of the Scientific Evidence on Associations Between Exposure to "Dampness" in Buildings and Health Effects). 2002. Indoor Air 15(10):7-16.

ORNL (Oak Ridge National Laboratory). 1988. The Building Foundation Design Handbook. ORNL/SUB/86-724143/1. Oak Ridge, TN: ORNL.

Phillips, R.W. 1997. Educational facility age and the academic achievement and attendance of upper elementary school students. Unpublished doctoral dissertation. Athens, GA: University of Georgia.

Phipatanakul, W., Cronin, B., Wood, R.A., Eggleston, P.A., Shih, M.C., Song, L., Tachdjian, R., and Oettgen, H.C. 2004. Effect of environmental intervention on mouse allergen levels in homes of inner-city Boston children with asthma. Ann. Allergy Asthma Immunol. 92(4):420-425.

Plumley, J.P., Jr. 1978. The impact of school building age on the academic achievement of pupils from selected schools in the state of Georgia. Unpublished doctoral dissertation. Athens, GA: University of Georgia.

Rea, M.S., ed. 2000. IESNA Lighting Handbook: Reference and Application. 9th edition. New York: Illuminating Engineering Society of North America.

Rea, M.S., and Bullough, J.D. 2001. Application efficacy. J. Illuminating Engineering Society 30(2):73-96.

Rea, M.S., and Ouellette, M.J. 1991. Relative visual performance: A basis for application. Light. Res. Technol. 23(3):135-144.

Rea, M.S., Ouellette, M.J., and Kennedy, M.E. 1985. Lighting and task parameters affecting posture, performance, and subjective ratings. J. Illuminating Engineering Society 15(1):231-238.

Rea, M.S., Figueiro, M.G., and Bullough, J.D. 2002. Circadian photobiology: An emerging framework for lighting practice and research. Light. Res. Technol. 34(3):177-190.

Reid, K.J., and Zee, P.C. 2004. Circadian rhythm disorders. Semin. Neurol. 24(3):315-325.

Rosen, L.N., Targum, S.D., Terman, M., Bryant, M.J., Hoffman, H., Kasper, S.F., Hamovit, J.R., Docherty, J.P., Welch, B., and Rosenthal, N.E. 1990. Prevalence of seasonal affective disorder at four latitudes. Psychiatry Res. 31(2):131-144.

Rosenthal, N. 1998. Winter Blues. Seasonal Affective Disorder. What It Is and How to Overcome It. New York and London: Guilford Press.

Rosenthal, N., Sack, D., Parry, B., Mendelsom, W., Tamarkin, L., and Wehr, T. 1985. Seasonal affective disorder and phototherapy. Ann. N.Y. Acad. Sci. 453:260.

Rusak, B., Eskes, G.A., and Shaw, S.R. 1997. Lighting and Human Health: A Review of the Literature. Ottawa: Canada Mortgage and Housing Corporation.

Satlin, A., Volicer, L., Ross, V., Herz, L., and Campbell, S. 1992. Bright light treatment of behavioral and sleep disturbances in patients with Alzheimer's disease. Am. J. Psychiatry 149:1028-1032.

Schneider, M. 2002. Public school facilities and teaching: Washington, DC, and Chicago. Available at www.edfacilities.org.

Schwartz, J. 2004. Air pollution and children's health. Pediatrics 113:1037-1043.

Seppanen, O.A., and Fisk, W.J. 2004. A model to estimate the cost effectiveness of indoor environment improvements in office work. Berkeley, CA: Lawrence Berkeley Laboratory.

Seppanen, O.A., and Fisk, W.J. 2005. Some quantitative relations between indoor environmental quality and work performance or health. Proceedings of Indoor Air 2005. Beijing, China.

Seppanen, O.A., Fisk, W.J., and Mendell, M.J. 1999. Association of ventilation rates and CO_2 concentrations with health and other human responses in commercial and institutional buildings. Indoor Air 9:226-252.

Shendell, D.G., Barnett, C., and Boese, S. 2004a. Science-based recommendations to prevent or reduce potential exposure to biological, chemical, and physical agents in schools. J. School Health 74(10):390-396.

Shendell, D.G., Prill, R., Fisk, W.J., Apte, M.G., Blake, O., and Faulkner, D. 2004b. Associations between classrooms' CO_2 concentrations and student attendance in Washington and Idaho. Indoor Air 14:333-341.

Slezak, J.A., Persky, V.W., Kuiz, F.J., and Byers, C. 1998. Asthama prevalence and risk factors in selected Head Start sites in Chicago, IL. J. Asthma 35:203-212.

Smedje, G., and Norbäck, D. 2000. New ventilation systems at select schools in Sweden—Effects on asthma and exposure. Arch. Environ. Health 55:18-25.

Stansfeld, S.A., Berglund, B., Clark., C., Lopez-Barrio, I., Fischer, P., Ohrstrom, E., Haines, M.M., Head, J., Hygge, S., van Kamp, I., and Berry, B.F. 2005. Aircraft and road traffic noise and children's cognition and health: A cross-national study. Lancet 365:1942-1949.

Stark, P.C., Burge, H.A., Ryan, L.M., Milton, D.K., and Gold, D.R. 2003. Fungal levels in the home and lower respiratory tract illnesses in the first year of life. Am. J. Resp. Crit. Care Med. 168:232-237.

Takaro, T.K., Krieger, J.W., and Song, L. 2004. Effect of environmental interventions to reduce exposure to asthma triggers in homes of low-income children in Seattle. J. Exposure Analysis Environ. Epidemiol. 14:S133-S143.

Thapan, K., Arendt, J., and Skene, D.J. 2001. An action spectrum for melatonin suppression: Evidence for a novel non-rod, non-cone photoreceptor system in humans. J. Physiol. 535:261-267.

Thomas, J.A. 1962. Efficiency in education: A study of the relationship between selected inputs and mean test scores in a sample of senior high schools. Unpublished doctoral dissertation. Palo Alto, CA: Stanford University.

Titze, I.R., Lemke, J., and Montequin, D. 1996. Populations in the U.S. workforce who rely on voice as a primary tool of trade. NCVS Status Progress Report 10:127-132.

Toftum, J., Jorgensen, A.S., and Fanger, P.O., 1998. Upper limits for air humidity to prevent warm respiratory discomfort. Energy and Buildings 28:15-23.

Turek, F.W., and Zee, P.C. 1999. Introduction to sleep and circadian rhythms. Pp. 1-17 in Turek, F.W., and Zee, P.C., eds., Regulation of Sleep and Circadian Rhythm. New York: Marcel Dekker.

Van Someren, E.J., Kessler, A., Mirmirann, M., and Swaab, D.F. 1997. Indirect bright light improves circadian rest-activity rhythm disturbances in demented patients. Biol. Psychiatry 41:955-963.

Wargocki, P., Sundell, J., Bischof, J., Brundrett, G., Fanger, P.O., Gyntelberg, F., Hanssen, O., Harrison, P., Pickering, A., Seppanen, O.A., and Wouters, P. 2002. Ventilation and health in non-industrial indoor environments: Report from European Multidisciplinary Scientific Consensus Meeting (EUROVEN). Indoor Air 12:113-128.

Wargocki, P., Wyon, D.P., Matysiak, B., and Irgens, S. 2005. The effects of classroom air temperature and outdoor air supply rate on the performance of school work by children. Proceedings of Indoor Air 2005. Beijing, China.

Weale, R.A. 1963. The Ageing Eye. London: HK Lewis and Company.

Weale, R.A. 1992. The Senescence of Human Vision. Oxford: Oxford University Press.

Williams, G.M., Linker, H.M., Waldvogel, M.G., Leidy, R.B., and Schal, C. 2005. Comparison of conventional and integrated pest management programs in public schools. J. Econ. Entomol. 98(4):1275-1283.

WSBE (Washington State Board of Education). 2005. Washington High Performance School Buildings: Report to the Legislature. Seattle, WA: Paladino and Company.

Wyon, D.P. 2004. The effects of indoor air quality on performance and productivity. Indoor Air 14(Suppl 7):92-101.

Appendix A

Biographies of Committee Members

John D. Spengler, Chair, is the Akira Yamaguchi Professor of Environmental Health and Human Habitation in the Department of Environmental Health at Harvard University's School of Public Health. He has conducted research in the areas of personal monitoring, air pollution health effects, aerosol characterization, indoor air pollution, and air pollution meteorology. More recently, he has been involved in research that includes the integration of knowledge about indoor and outdoor air pollution as well as other risk factors into the design of housing, buildings, and communities. He uses the tools of life-cycle analysis, risk assessment, and activity-based costing as indicators to measure the sustainable attributes of alternative designs, practices, and community development. He serves as adviser to the World Health Organization on indoor air pollution, personal exposure, and air pollution epidemiology, and he has served as either a member or consultant on various U.S. EPA Science Advisory Board committees. He received a B.S. in physics from the University of Notre Dame, an M.S. in environmental health sciences from Harvard University, and a Ph.D. in atmospheric sciences from the State University of New York-Albany.

Vivian E. Loftness, Vice Chair, is a professor of architecture at Carnegie Mellon University. She is an international energy and building performance consultant for commercial and residential building design and has researched and written extensively on energy conservation, passive solar design, climate, and regionalism in architecture. Professor Loftness has worked for many years with the Architectural and Building Sciences Division of Public Works Canada, researching and developing the issues of total building performance and the field of building diagnostics. Through the Advanced Building Systems Integration Consortium, she has been actively researching and designing high-performance office environments. Professor Loftness is a member of the advisory board at Johnson Controls and Owens-Corning Fiberglass Construction. She has been involved in international organizations including as resident, Executive Interchange Canada Architecture and Building Sciences, Department of Public Works Canada (October 1982 to June 1985) and as principal investigator, World Meteorological Organization, for Climate/Energy Graphics, and she has previously served on NRC committees. She holds a B.S. in architecture and a master's of architecture from the Massachusetts Institute of Technology.

Charlene W. Bayer is the Research Institute Branch head, principal research scientist, and adjunct professor at the Georgia Institute of Technology. A reviewer for the *Journal of Chromatographic Science, Indoor Air,* and *Analytical and Bioanalytical Chemistry,* and periodically for a variety of other peer-reviewed journals and conference proceedings, she has expertise in indoor environments, air quality, and related health concerns. Dr. Bayer is a past member of the ASHRAE Environmental Health Committee and serves on numerous other review committees for Underwriters' Laboratories, the U.S. Environmental Protection

Agency, Oak Ridge National Laboratory, and the American Chemical Society. Dr. Bayer was a semifinalist in *Discovery Magazine* awards for Innovative Technology of Importance in 1999 and holds numerous patents for materials and devices for monitoring and improving air quality. Her current research includes a project to develop a personal monitoring vest able to monitor a variety of pollutants that are suspected as being asthmatic aggravators while linking these with pulmonary function tests sponsored by the Department of Housing and Urban Development. She holds a B.S. in chemistry form Baylor University and an M.S. and a Ph.D. in organic chemistry from Emory University.

John S. Bradley is a principal research officer at the National Research Council of Canada's Institute for Research in Construction. Dr. Bradley is involved in the design of efficient procedures for making advanced acoustical measurements in rooms for speech and music, and the use of these quantities to evaluate such spaces more scientifically; measuring techniques for predicting and evaluating speech intelligibility in rooms, including school classrooms; noise control related to buildings, including for outdoor noises; and relationships between physical and subjective assessments of annoyance caused by noise from various sources. He is a fellow in the Acoustical Society of America, past president of the Canadian Acoustical Association, and a member of the Acoustical Society of America Technical Committee on Architectural Acoustics and the editorial board of the Audio Engineering Society. He has served on ANSI and ISO standards committees as well as the WHO working group for community noise guidelines. He holds a B.S. in physics and a master's in physics/acoustics from the University of Western Ontario, and a Ph.D. in physics/acoustics from Imperial College, University of London.

Glen I. Earthman is professor emeritus of educational administration at Virginia Polytechnic Institute and State University. His research interests extend to all phases of school facilities, with a concentration on exploring the relationship between school building condition and student achievement. Dr. Earthman has 40 years of experience in the field of education, serving as a teacher, principal, and executive director for school facility planning in the Philadelphia public schools, where he directed a staff of 250 professional planners and architects engaged in all activities associated with planning school facilities and monitoring the construction and evaluation of the resultant buildings. He is a member and past officer of the International Society for Educational Planning and the Council of Educational Facility Planners, International (CEFPI). He received the CEFPI President's Award for planning activities in 1992 and the Planner of the Year Award in 1994. He holds a B.A. and a master's degree from the University of Denver and a Ph.D. from the University of Northern Colorado, where he served as a graduate fellow in the School Planning Laboratory.

Peyton A. Eggleston is the director of the Center for Children's Environmental Health at Johns Hopkins University, a center of excellence sponsored by the National Institute of Environmental Health Sciences and one of EPA's National Centers for Environmental Research. He is also a professor of pediatrics at the Johns Hopkins School of Medicine. His research focus is environmental allergens—their role in respiratory diseases (in particular, asthma), risk factors for sensitization, means of avoidance, and methods and effectiveness of indoor environmental control. He is credited with more than 190 publications and serves on the editorial board of the *Journal of Allergy and Clinical Immunology*. He has served as a member of the Board of Allergy and Immunology and is an active member of the Academy of Asthma, Allergy, and Immunology. Dr. Eggleston received his medical degree from the University of Virginia and training in pediatrics and allergy-immunology at the University of Washington.

Paul Fisette is the director and an associate professor of building materials and wood technology and an associate professor of architecture at the University of Massachusetts, Amherst. Professor Fisette's research and professional focus involve the performance of building systems, energy-efficient construction, sustainable building practices, and the performance of building materials. He has developed an innovative Web service that provides technical advice on the performance, specification, and use of building materials. Professor Fisette has written more than 200 published works on building science and construction technology. Previous to his current position, he owned and operated a general contracting business and was a senior editor with *Custom Builder Magazine,* covering technical information and innovations of interest to small- and medium-sized residential building firms. Professor Fisette is a member of the National Research Council's Board on Infrastructure and the Constructed Environment (BICE) and a contributing editor for the *Journal of Light Construction,* and he has served on a variety of editorial and professional advisory boards. He holds B.S. and M.S. degrees in wood science and technology from the University of Massachusetts.

Caroline Breese Hall, M.D., is a professor of pediatrics and medicine in infectious diseases at the University of Rochester School of Medicine. At Rochester her research has focused on virology, especially respiratory syncytial virus, human herpes virus 6, and vaccines, resulting in more than 500 published articles. Among the national positions Dr. Hall has held are president of the Pediatric Infectious Diseases Society; member of the Red Book Committee for 8 years and chairman for 4 years; and member of the CDC's Advisory Committee of Immunization Practices, the Board of Scientific Counselors for the National Center of Infectious Diseases, committees for the Institute of Medicine, the American Board for Pediatric Infectious Diseases, and the Subboard for Pediatric Infectious Diseases. Among the awards she has received are the Pediatric Infectious Diseases Society Distinguished Physician Award and the Clinical Virology Award from the Pan American Society of Virology, as well as being named among the best doctors in America and among the top 20 women physicians in America. She graduated from Wellesely College and Rochester Medical School and did her subsequent residency training at Yale, followed by fellowships first in pediatric infectious diseases and then allergy and immunology in the Department of Medicine at Yale University.

Gary T. Henry is a professor of policy studies in the Andrew Young School of Policy Studies at Georgia State University, where he specializes in educational policy, school accountability, and program evaluation. He previously served as the director of evaluation and learning services for the David and Lucile Packard Foundation. Dr. Henry has evaluated a variety of policies and programs, including pre-K and the HOPE Scholarship program in Georgia as well as school reforms and accountability systems. He has served as the director of the university's Applied Research Center. He is the author of *Practical Sampling* (Sage 1990) and *Graphing Data* (Sage 1995) and co-author of *Evaluation: An Integrated Framework for Understanding, Guiding, and Improving Policies and Programs* (Jossey-Bass

2000), and he has published extensively in the field of evaluation and policy analysis. In addition, he served as deputy secretary of education for the Commonwealth of Virginia and chief methodologist with the Joint Legislative Audit and Review Commission for the Virginia General Assembly. He received the Evaluation of the Year Award from the American Evaluation Association in 1998 for his work with Georgia's Council for School Performance and the Joseph Wholey Distinguished Scholarship Award in 2001 from the American Society for Public Administration and the Center for Accountability and Performance. He received his Ph.D. from the University of Wisconsin.

Clifford S. Mitchell is an associate professor and director of the Occupational Medicine Residency Program at the Johns Hopkins Bloomberg School of Public Health. His research interests include indoor air quality and its effects on human health in schools and in office buildings. He holds a B.A. from Williams College, an M.S. from the Massachusetts Institute of Technology, an M.D. from Case Western Reserve, and an M.P.H. from Johns Hopkins University School of Public Health.

Mark S. Rea is the director of the Lighting Research Center at Rensselaer Polytechnic Institute (RPI), a position he has held since 1988. He is also a professor at the School of Architecture and in the Department of Philosophy, Psychology, and Cognitive Science at RPI. Prior to RPI he was the manager of the Indoor Environment Program, Building Performance Section at the National Research Council of Canada. He also has been a visiting scientist at the Electricity Council Research Centre, Capenhurst, United Kingdom. He is a fellow of the Illuminating Engineering Society of North America and of the Society of Light and Lighting (United Kingdom). He is on the international editorial advisory board of the *Lighting Research and Technology Journal* and is editor-in-chief of the *Illuminating Engineering Society of North America Lighting Handbook* (8th and 9th editions). He received the William H. Wiley Distinguished Faculty Award from RPI and the Gold Medal from the Illuminating Engineering Society of North America. Dr. Rea received a B.S. in psychology and an M.S. and a Ph.D. in biophysics from Ohio State University.

Henry Sanoff is professor emeritus of architecture at the North Carolina State University College of Design. He came to the College of Design in 1966 from the University of California, Berkeley, where he was an assistant professor. He is a member of the Academy of Outstanding Teachers and has been designated an Alumni Distinguished Graduate Professor. Mr. Sanoff teaches courses related to community participation, social architecture, design research, design methodology, and design programming. He has been a visiting lecturer and scholar at more than 85 institutions in the United States and abroad. He is the U.S. editor of *The Journal of Design Studies* and a member of the editorial board of the *Journal of Architecture and Planning Research.* Professor Sanoff is also recognized as one of the founders of the Environmental Design Research Association (EDRA) in 1969. His research has concentrated on the areas of social housing, children's environments, community arts, aging populations, and community participation. Professor Sanoff received a bachelor of architecture and a master of architecture from Pratt Institute.

Carol H. Weiss is the Beatrice B. Whiting Professor of Education at the Harvard Graduate School of Education, where she teaches in the areas of administration, planning, and social policy. Her courses include evaluation methods, research methods, use of research as a strategy for change, and organizational decision making. She has published 11 books, 3 of which are on evaluation and 5 on the uses of research and evaluation in policy making. Her recent work is about the influences on educational policy making exerted by information, ideology, interests, information, and institutional constraints. She has been a fellow at the Center for Advanced Study in the Behavioral Sciences, a guest scholar at the Brookings Institution, a congressional fellow under the sponsorship of the American Sociological Association, a senior fellow at the U.S. Department of Education, and a member of seven panels of the National Academy of Sciences. She is on editorial boards for the *Teachers College Record*, *Journal of Educational Change, Journal of Comparative Policy Analysis, Asia-Pacific Journal of Teacher Education and Development, American Behavioral Scientist*, and others. She holds a Ph.D. in sociology from Columbia University.

Suzanne M. Wilson is a professor of teacher education in the Department of Teacher Education Michigan State University. She is an educational psychologist with an interest in teacher learning and teacher knowledge. Her studies include the capacities and commitment of exemplary secondary school history and mathematics teachers, and she has written extensively on the knowledge base of teaching. She recently concluded a longitudinal study of the relationship between educational policy and teaching practice by examining efforts to reform mathematics teaching in California. She is also the director of the Center for the Scholarship of Teaching. Her areas of expertise include curriculum policy, history of teachers and teaching, mathematics reform, teacher assessment, teacher education and learning, and teaching history. Dr. Wilson earned her Ph.D. from Stanford University.

Role of the Board on Infrastructure and the Constructed Environment

The Board on Infrastructure and the Constructed Environment (BICE) was established by the National Research Council (NRC) in 1946 as the Building Research Advisory Board. BICE and its predecessor organizations have been the principal units of the NRC concerned with the relationship between the constructed and natural environments and their interaction with human activities. Principal areas of focus include:

- Human factors and the built environment,
- Project management methods,
- Construction methods and materials,
- Security of facilities and critical infrastructure,
- Multihazard mitigation methods,
- Construction and utilization of underground space, and
- Infrastructure and community building.

The BICE brings together experts from a wide range of scientific, engineering, and social science disciplines to discuss potential studies of interest; develop and frame study tasks; ensure proper project planning; suggest possible reviewers for reports produced by fully independent ad hoc study committees; and convene meetings to examine strategic issues. The board members listed in the front of this document were not asked to endorse the committee's conclusions or recommendations, nor did they see the final draft of this report before its release.

Additional information about the BICE can be obtained online at http://www.nationalacademies.org/bice.

We Spoke Jewish

Yiddishkeit

Fingers fly,
Hands gesture,
Passion ill-contained
In Midwestern strictures.
We are a high-energy people.
We speak quickly,
Seldom waiting for a sentence to end
To interject.
We express and emote.
Through jokes and gesture
We occupy space.
Yiddishkeit
Spilling from our fingertips.

Yiddishkeit is energy and language,
Everything
And every day,
A waterfall of words,
We are built for expression,
Not containment,
And words,
Words of action,
Tzedakah, Mitzvah,
Natural words and natural things,
Things we make happen,
We are a people
Called to act.

—Susan Weinberg
inspired by an interview with Fannie Schanfield

We Spoke Jewish

A LEGACY IN STORIES

Text and Artwork by Susan Weinberg

Published by the Jewish Historical Society of the Upper Midwest
Minneapolis, Minnesota

This publication was made possible in part by the people of Minnesota through a grant funded by an appropriation to the Minnesota Historical Society from the Minnesota Arts & Cultural Heritage Fund. Any views, findings, opinions, conclusions or recommendations expressed in this publication are those of the authors and do not necessarily represent those of the State of Minnesota, the Minnesota Historical Society, or the Minnesota Historic Resources Advisory Committee.

The Jewish Historical Society of the Upper Midwest can be contacted at the Eloise and Elliot Kaplan History Center, Jay and Rose Phillips Building, Barry Family Campus, 4330 S. Cedar Lake Road, Minneapolis, MN 55416. E-mail history@jhsum.org

JEWISH HISTORICAL SOCIETY
of the Upper Midwest

Printed in the United States of America

ISBN 978-0-9993106-0-1

Cover Art: *From Her Mother* by Susan Weinberg, wespokejewish.com

Dedication

To my mother, Rose Weinberg,
who bequeathed to me her love of art, history, and story,
and taught me to listen with my heart.

Her presence was deeply felt throughout.

Table of Contents

A Legacy of Story ix

The Interviews ix

The Artwork xi

Speaking Jewish xii

A Foot in Both Worlds 1

Shirley Sussman 3

Old World Customs 3

The Lyndale Shul 4

We Spoke Only Jewish 6

Bernice Cowl Gordon 9

Stumping the Teacher 9

Fannie Schanfield 11

Yiddishkeit 11

A Legacy of Storytelling 12

Zelda Katz 17

A Legacy of Relationship 17

Anne Milavetz 19

Sharing Traditions 19

Dorothy Brochin Wittcoff 23

Body and Soul 23

Helping Those in Need 24

An Adventurous Life 25

Harold Wittcoff 27

The Second Jew 27

A Few Thoughts 30

Of Loss and Survival 31

Hanna Lyon 33

The Kindertransport 33

Trudy Rappaport 37

Stuck in Germany 37

Postcard from New Ulm 40

Sam Saide 43

Living by His Wits 43

Walter Schwarz 47

A Narrow Escape 47

A Ritchie Boy 48

A Few Thoughts 50

Jews from the USSR 51

Rakhil Sheynkman 53

A History Lesson 53

A War Hero 54

Becoming a Citizen 55

Food, Song, and Story 56

Secondhand Kind of Person 57

Boris Lerner 61

A Child Survivor 61

Yevgeniy Mazo 65

Unchained Legacy 65

A Few Thoughts 68

The Living Archive 69
Antisemitism 69
Community 71
Immigration 73

Legacy: The Next Generation 77

Final Thoughts 81

Acknowledgments 83
Author Biography 85
Glossary 87
Paintings by Susan Weinberg 91
Bibliography 93
Interviews 93
Other Sources 93
Notes 97
Index 99
About my Partners 101

A Legacy of Story

The Interviews

This project happened by chance. In 2010, I was meeting with staff at Sholom, a Twin Cities Jewish residential facility for elders. I wanted to explore their interest in exhibiting art I had created based on stories from my own family history. As we talked back and forth about my artwork, it suddenly occurred to me that Sholom itself was filled with stories. It was home to many Jewish elders who were long-time members of the Jewish community, each with a story to tell. Collectively, they represent part of a larger community legacy. Impulsively, I blurted out, "Wouldn't it be interesting if I could interview residents and develop artwork around *their* stories?"

This thought, once expressed, soon took on life. Sholom staff shared my enthusiasm, and before long I was meeting with the rabbi and program staff to explore how this could become a reality. Often, I heard, "Oh, if only you could have done this ten years ago," as staff expressed dismay at all the stories that had been lost. I was still able to capture a small segment of the stories that have passed through Sholom and the broader Jewish community, a segment so rich that I, too, have often wished I could turn back the clock and collect more.

To some extent, this project has been an exploration of my own interest in Jewish identity as a secular Jew. I strongly identify with being Jewish, but I have not been religious in practice and for many years was not active in the Jewish community. Where does this sense of identity come from? What does it mean? Identity was my initial focus, at least in part because of questions about my own identity.

So why does identity matter? Studies have found that children who know about their family history are more emotionally healthy and better able to recover from difficult challenges. It's all about having a unifying narrative. Robyn Fivish, Jennifer Bohanek, and Marshall Duke, colleagues at Emory's Center for Myth and Ritual in American Life, found it is through reminiscing and family stories that children develop an "intergenerational self," defining their place within a larger family narrative. It is by anchoring their sense of self in a broader family context that they become strengthened.

These researchers report that stories of the past provide a framework that helps us to make sense of our own experiences.

We construct a sense of self through time that relies both on an evaluative perspective of our own personal history, as well as how our history fits into larger cultural and historical frameworks. We are who we are because of what we have experienced and what we have been told; our sense of self is constructed from both personal history and the social cultural history in which our personal history is embedded.[1]

I began to wonder if this same principle could be true of a community, helping to strengthen our sense of community and our place within it.

Early on, I realized the remarkable depth of the stories I encountered and the many ways they could be shared. My initial purpose in using narratives to create artwork broadened to include storytelling through video and text as well. Originally recording the interviews to create a record for reference, I soon realized there was value in sharing excerpts of the videos themselves, enriching the elders' stories with their own words, their own voices. My project continued to grow. Story was still at its center, now told in multiple ways.

In my first set of interviews with the elders, I attempted to get a mix of people across three groups:

- First-generation Americans raised in Minnesota's early Jewish communities,
- Holocaust survivors who immigrated in the 1940s and 50s, and
- Refugees from the former Soviet Union who arrived in the 1970s and later.

While those in the first-generation group were not immigrants themselves, they grew up in an immigrant culture and represented the immigrant experience of their parents and communities. Holocaust survivors and refugees from the former Soviet Union had first-hand immigrant experiences.

In addition to Sholom, I collaborated with the Jewish Historical Society of the Upper Midwest (JHSUM) and then brought in storyteller Carla Vogel to assist in the interviews. Sholom is composed of several Twin Cities campuses that offer a continuum of care. Our interviews included all of the campuses, covering elders who lived independently as well as those in nursing home facilities.

When these interviews were completed, I stopped by the office of the JHSUM to share some video segments with the director. As I was basking in the satisfaction of having completed this project, one that had grown far beyond what I had originally envisioned, she offered a suggestion, "If this is about legacy, what about interviewing their children?" Apparently, I wasn't done yet!

A second grant focused on children and grandchildren, exploring legacy that had been passed down. Half of these families included elders I had already interviewed. Now, with the younger generations, we would build on the stories they had shared. The elder was present for each of these interviews, so there was an interplay between family members, each drawing out stories from the other.

The other half were completely new families. Not only were we gathering these stories for the first time, but now we were also including children and grandchildren. There were a lot of voices to capture, even as we were first learning each new story. This presented several challenges, some as basic as fitting everyone into the framing of the video camera.

Another challenge of this project was the age of my interviewees. Most were in their 90s when we did the initial interviews in 2011 and 2012. By the time I began this book several years later, the aging process had often limited the possibility of returning to build out the stories in different ways. I needed to work with what I already had.

Interviewing immigrants from the former Soviet Union was challenging because of the language barrier. These interviews were done with the aid of a translator, sometimes a staff member of Sholom or a family member, and are edited for translation. Despite the language barrier, I was struck by how much could be conveyed through gesture and expression. Each interviewee had a distinct personality that came through clearly, even without a common language.

Over the course of this project, I came to a deep appreciation of my interviewees. I was struck by how articulate and forceful many proved to be. They were strong personalities, often outspoken individuals and extraordinary storytellers. Others were deceptively soft-spoken as they related difficult challenges that had required considerable courage to confront. We live in a culture that often dismisses elders as no longer offering anything of value, yet these individuals lived full lives, and they made an impact on the world, continuing to influence those with whom they came in contact.

The Artwork

When I completed the interviews, I turned to the artwork. I had thought this would be the easy part. I soon discovered it required many decisions. How was I going to tell these stories in paint? At first, I considered portraits. So often a series on elders focuses on how they appear today, but my focus was on story, and stories happen throughout a lifetime. I decided to do portraits only if they were important to the story. While portraits can be found throughout this series, some are of a subject's mother or father or sibling; others are of my interviewee at a much younger age, as I pictured them in my imagination.

Before painting, I would reread the interview transcript, then set it aside and do something totally unrelated. Parts of the interview would bubble up in my mind, and that's how my paintings began to evolve. It was those stories that rose to the top that would become my material, typically those that were visual or emotional, or offered surprising new information. The interviews were not dry histories, but vivid perspectives on an individual's life experience. They contained the nuances that bring history to life and create a new and deeper understanding.

Studies have found that people who read good literature have a greater level of empathy because of the need to imagine themselves in the story.[2] Artwork like this requires similar empathy. To paint someone's story, I must experience it on a level of deep feeling. I imagined what it felt like to pull myself back in fear as chickens next to the bed cackled at me. I pictured myself polishing the fireplace as I swallowed the pit in my stomach, feeling something terrible has happened to my family. It is hard for me to listen to someone's story and not feel a connection. It is impossible to paint it and not consider their underlying feelings.

Each painting was a discovery, a story whose center I had to find. Some stories were more laden with emotion and hence easier to imagine and paint. Often I found my way in by writing poetry from the perspective of my interviewees, imagining their experiences on both physical and emotional levels. What started as word pictures led to visual imagery that formed a painting.

Other stories drew me in by revealing information that was new to me. For example, I had known nothing of the houses abandoned by Germans, where some Jews found refuge upon being freed. Nor had I heard of the Nazi sale of bricks from the Warsaw ghetto to local Poles. I didn't know the significance of "line 5" on the former Russian passport, marking one as Jewish, or that "acting Jewish" included using one's hands to gesture while speaking. It is no surprise these are the stories I chose to represent in my artwork, for they included the element of discovery, which inspires creation.

Speaking Jewish

The three groups who were interviewed came from three distinct segments of the Jewish community. In the late 19th and early 20th century, a wave of Jewish immigrants came from Eastern Europe, fleeing *pogroms* and poverty. Newcomers clustered together, and synagogues sprang up to serve those arriving from common geographic areas. This group that grew up in Minnesota often had warm memories of their former Jewish communities. They spoke of family shops, Jewish institutions, and helping each other in times of need. Several sang songs for us. Some shared artifacts that had legacy embedded within them.

Holocaust survivors and the later Jewish refugees from the Soviet Union were grafted onto this community. The survivors had stories of loss, loss of family and community and the lives they had lived prior to the war. They also had stories of survival in the face of loss. The Jews from the Soviet Union had stories of antisemitism, of existing as a "secondhand kind of person," of raising their children in a world that imposed limitations on them solely because they were Jewish.

The phrase "speaking Jewish" is often used to describe using the *Yiddish* language, and in the community of Eastern European Jews who lived in Minnesota in the 1920s, virtually everyone spoke Jewish. While many survivors and some Soviet immigrants spoke Yiddish, many also spoke Jewish in different ways.

Survivors spoke the Jewish of remembrance, carrying with them the memory of once-thriving Jewish communities and the people who populated them. Their stories, their memories, keep the history of those communities alive. They also play an important role in preserving the memory of the Holocaust and its lessons for future generations.

Immigrants from the former Soviet Union could not openly practice Judaism, but they carried their Jewish heritage forward nonetheless. They spoke Jewish to their children through story, song, and food, keeping their Judaism alive through culture. All three groups who lent their voices to this book spoke Jewish, albeit in different ways. Collectively they represent our language, memory, and culture, all vehicles that convey important aspects of Jewish identity.

While many of those I interviewed displayed a clear identity associated with the Jewish religion, others' Jewish identity was shaped by the exclusion and persecution they had known. Some were very religious, others secular. For many it was the sense of community within their synagogue that was an important part of their Jewish experience. For others, Jewish identity was defined by early exposure to Jewish traditions, either carried forward throughout their lives or rediscovered later in life.

Some talked about being Jewish, about the freedom to be Jewish in the United States. Others described legacy in terms of embracing *Yiddishkeit*, the Jewish culture, and integrating it into their lives. They also talked about the legacies they had been given and which they themselves carried forward in telling the stories, parenting the children, and honoring the parents.

As this project unfolded, I recognized that even my family members who came over in the early 1900s could just as easily have stayed in Europe and given birth to those who became survivors of the Holocaust or immigrants from the USSR in the late twentieth century. Our early story was the same, with the trajectory only altered by *when* our families came to the United States. My perch of relative safety in the world easily could have been something quite different.

My most startling shock of recognition came during an interview with an immigrant from the Ukraine. What had started feeling arm's length suddenly became uncomfortably close, as he told me that my ancestral town was the place where his aunt and cousin were shot. I wondered what family of mine had shared that fate.

These stories are often visually rich, and the storytellers often relished their retelling. Some of the stories are painful. Many are deeply moving. A few clearly articulate identity and legacy. More often they are stories from which legacy and identity emerge, not neatly packaged, but evident nonetheless. Collectively they represent many of the life experiences that create Jewish identity and the legacy of our broader community.

A Foot in Both Worlds

Interviewees born during the period that spanned World War I, grew up in an immigrant community that was predominantly Jewish. Typically, their parents were immigrants, as were many of their neighbors. The largest concentration of these Jews had been on the North Side of Minneapolis, which by 1936 was home to two-thirds of the Minneapolis Jewish community.[3] Smaller communities were found on the South Side of Minneapolis and the West Side of St. Paul. Antisemitism was a dominant force in the United States, and especially in Minneapolis, well into the first half of the twentieth century. This influenced employment, housing, and immigration. Hiring barriers in the larger community meant that many in this group had grown up with immigrant parents who ran stores to serve their Jewish neighbors. They were surrounded by people who spoke Yiddish, with the children often interpreting in family dealings with the English-speaking world. Old World customs were common. The first generation born in the United States faced an underlying pressure to fit into American culture. Often that was understood as "not acting Jewish."

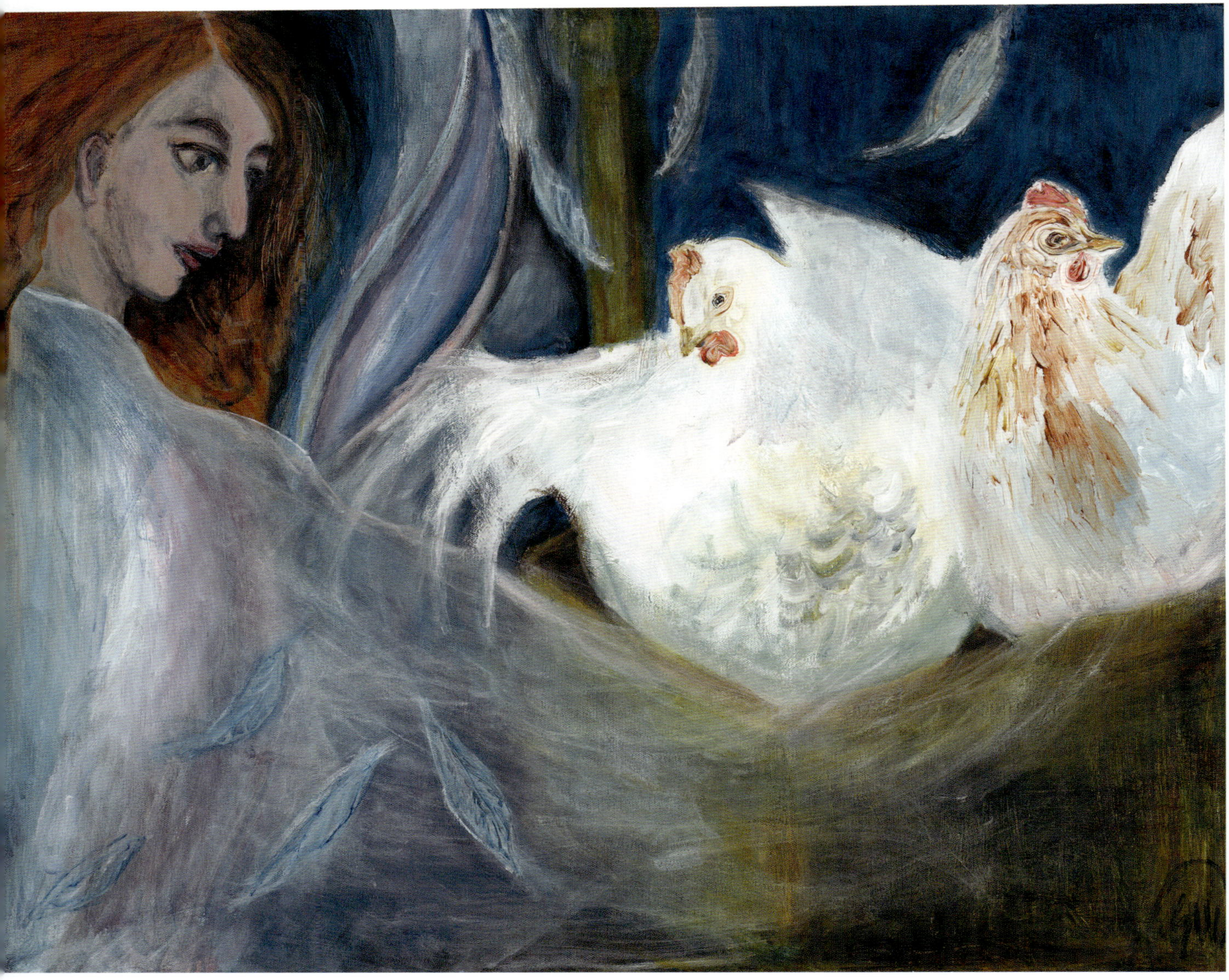

Sleeping with the Chickens, from the story of Shirley Sussman

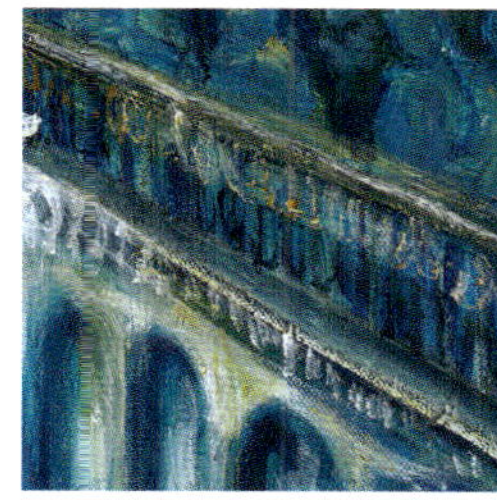

Shirley Sussman

Old World Customs

Even as she leaned over her walker, I could see that Shirley Sussman was a tall woman, and I guessed that as a young woman she carried herself with a certain elegance. She had a long face crowned with red hair, and she had energy, an energy I often see in good storytellers. As she spoke, she occupied her story, stepping into it through a child's eyes, reliving it in her retelling. Her words came in a rush, and her presence filled the room.

Shirley remembered her visits to her grandmother's house with no great fondness, due to the sleeping arrangement:

> *I remember . . . after I was born that we lived on Emerson also . . . When my Aunt Tillie, my grandmother's . . . daughter, when she decided to take a vacation . . . to go up to Wisconsin to see her sister, they didn't want my grandmother to live alone. So, who do they pick to go live with my grandmother? Me . . .*
>
> *I remember . . . my grandmother had a one-bedroom apartment. It was upstairs . . . She had a mattress—must have been about that thick* [holds hands a few feet apart] *all feathers, you know—and a stool to get up.*
>
> *Time to go to bed, I crawled in to get into bed to sleep with her . . . Next to the bed my grandmother had two live chickens in a box, and I was deathly afraid of chickens, and that's where I had to sleep that night, with the live chickens there . . .*
>
> *She'd* [later] *go to the* shoykhet *. . . and have the chickens killed. She'd carry them to the shoykhet and come back and* flick *them. Sit in the back yard and flick 'em. Every time on a weekend. She'd go, like, on a Friday morning before Shabbos started and get her chickens, and when I'd come to sleep with her, she'd have the chickens Friday. And every time I went, I had to go sleep there, and I had to sleep with those chickens. I'll never forget that. I was scared to death.*

Can you picture Shirley, locking her gaze with the beady eyes of those chickens? This was the first painting I did in the series because I could picture it so easily. I imagined Shirley as a young woman with her long face and red hair, nervously watching the chickens. I decided the gaze between Shirley and one chicken was the focal point, and I extended the bedcovers in a line to echo that. I made the feathers of one chicken look rather menacing, and then I let the feathers fly!

The Lyndale Shul

Synagogues were important institutions in the community, often serving those who came from the same country. Shirley Sussman remembered her visits to the old Lyndale Shul through a child's eyes. It was an impressive building, and her perspective was from the women's balcony.

> *We went to the old* shul *on Lyndale, the Lyndale Shul. That was a beautiful building. It was just gorgeous. It really was the prettiest one, I think, ever built in this whole state. It had the columns. When you walked in there, you felt you were in a shul, you were in a house of worship. You weren't just in a fancy place where this one had candy and this one was serving . . . No, you went to a shul. And of course, the women sat upstairs. I sat upstairs with my mother. And I don't know how anybody would pray there, because everybody was talking to somebody else, kissing all the kids and talking to someone else . . .*
>
> *A week before the holidays they'd have a late service until 11 o'clock at night. It was always later with the Orthodox shuls because they had more to say. It always took later than it said so in the book. They had more to read, they had more to say, then they would stop, and then they would talk to somebody here and talk to somebody there, and then they'd stand there with a big gavel and say,* 'Lozn sha.' *You know, people would talk, so then they would say 'Lozn sha.' Well, so that's what they did, so we didn't get home until late. The kids, a lot of us—I was a kid then, and my mother would give me her coat, and I'd cover up and lay down on the empty seats around there and sleep until they were through. My father would carry me home.*

As I imagined the shul, I thought of the women's balcony as a unique world, separate and distinct from the realm of men. In my painting, I wanted this space to be defined, while the world of the men below was blurred and indistinct. I pictured it from a child's perspective, being lulled to sleep by voices. Shirley dozes off with her mother's hand resting lightly upon her, creating a sense of safety and security.

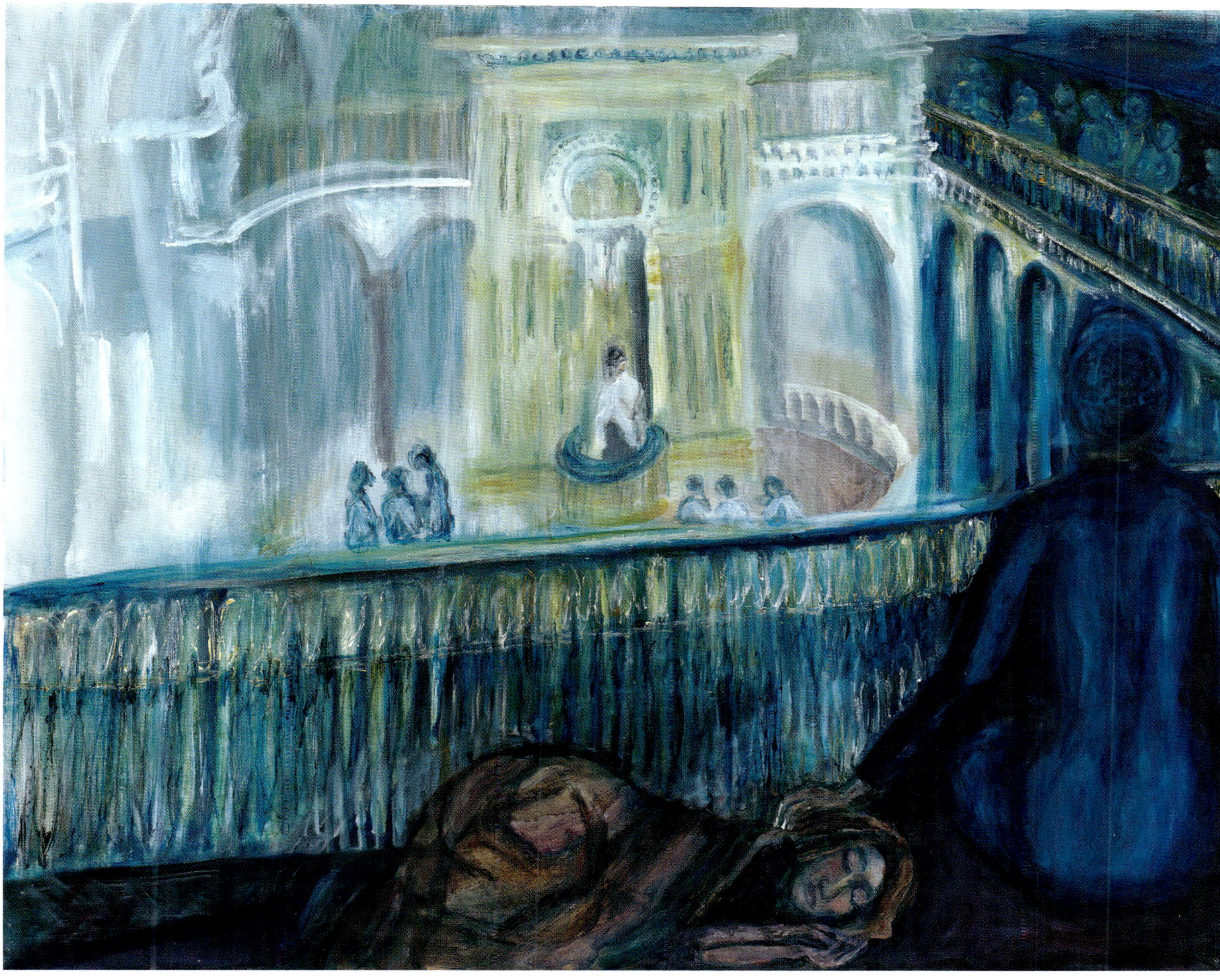

Lozn Sha, from the story of Shirley Sussman

We Spoke Only Jewish

Shirley's father had a butcher shop on Girard and 6th Avenue. Some responsibility came with that role. Shirley recalled her father assisting families in need:

> *My father, when it came a holiday . . . there were families, big families, and they were very, very poor. Their husbands either were junk peddlers or they weren't working at all . . . and so when come the holidays, my father was always making packages . . . my father would take some of the kids that lived there for* yontif. *He'd take them to Sam Bass on Lyndale and 6th Avenue North and buy them shoes for the holidays.*

Stores were often family affairs, and Shirley learned how to help at her father's shop. All the business and records were conducted in Yiddish, "Jewish," as Shirley called it:

> *And we spoke only Jewish. Only. There was no such thing as not speaking Jewish. And then my father had the meat market, and you know everything in his meat market, all his books—books that people had orders, every customer had a book with their name in it—everything was written in Jewish, you see.*
>
> *I would help in the butcher shop. I started to help in there when I was ten or eleven years old. I knew all the customers. I spoke Jewish when they came in, to them . . . and I would write in English in their book, and then I would tell my father, and he'd translate it into Jewish, so he'd know what was on there.*

Shirley remembered they spoke only Yiddish at home, except for her older brother who was more a part of the outside world. He spoke English but understood Yiddish. She recalled how her father learned English at the school where she went to kindergarten:

> *Years ago, there was the Sumner School . . . It was between Colfax, Bryant, and Lyndale. There was a big school on the side of 6th Avenue North. The school was on the ground, no grass, it was just sand around it. In the front of the school, they had these little white huts where they had separate classes there. That's where my father went to learn how to read English and to write English. I would go for kindergarten. He would go to learn to read English. When I got to school, it was different. I talked English. In fact, my mother used to say, 'Talk English,' and so I did.*

Like many children of immigrant families, Shirley straddled two worlds. Family, community, and shul immersed Shirley in the Old World heritage of the Jewish immigrant community. At home she spoke Jewish, yet she learned to step into another world by speaking English at school and later as her parents' translator when necessary. Still, in the store, in the neighborhood, and in her home, Jewish was the dominant language.

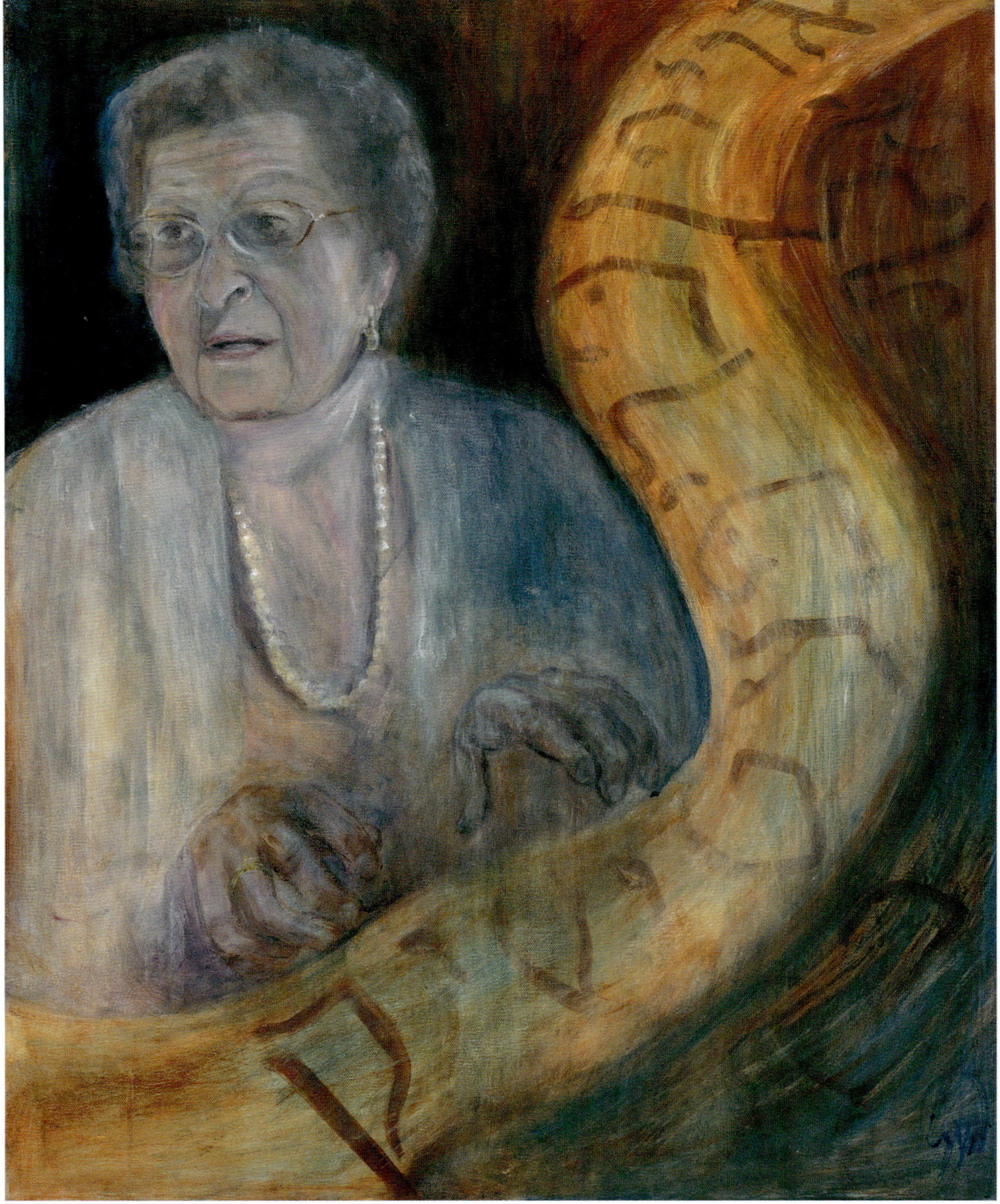

Alef-Beys, from the story of Bernice Gordon

Bernice Cowl Gordon

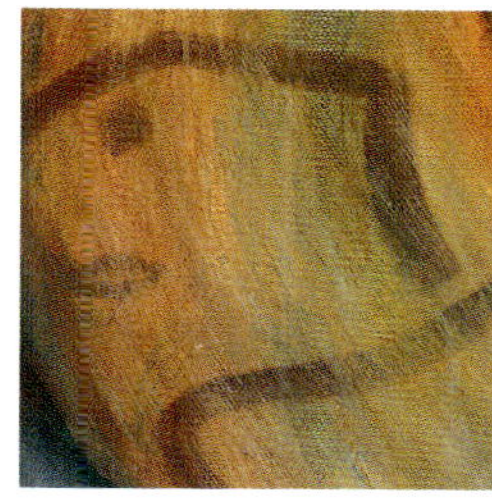

Stumping the Teacher

Today Yiddish is still spoken by those who grew up in the early Jewish community, but the number of speakers has diminished. It is taught at Sholom, where Bernice Cowl Gordon attended classes well into her 90s. Bernice had a unique style. She took care with her appearance, well dressed in a white jacket with pink blouse and pearls. She had an air of mischief and a girlish giggle that punctuated her conversation.

When we asked her what she liked about Yiddish she replied,

> *There's a lot of power in Yiddish, a lot of fire . . .*
>
> *Just before you came in, I was resting my eyes, and I was thinking about what new word could I bring to the Yiddish class that's tomorrow . . . I'm always thinking of things that could stump the teacher . . .*
>
> Kasokeh, *did you ever hear of that? . . . It's 'cross-eyed.'*
>
> *There's another word . . .* zahike. *That's 'somebody who stutters.'*
>
> *There's one more I thought of . . . but I won't tell it to them all in one day. It's hard to think of new words that she doesn't know.*

"How would you say someone was a cross-eyed stutterer?" I asked.

> Ich ben a kasokeh zahike mensch.
>
> *One more:* kalamutne. *Kalamutne means—it doesn't mean 'sad' and it doesn't mean 'depressed'—it means something in between.*

There was a wit to many of Bernice's stories, and she laughed freely as she retold them. Her mischievous humor shined through as she described the colorful Yiddish words her Uncle Herschel would use while driving. Well, it is a colorful language!

We asked her how she thought about her Jewish identity, and she replied, "There is something very strong-minded and stiff-necked about being Jewish. When you're Jewish you are just Jewish, and that's all there is."

Bernice had a beautiful singing voice and sang for us the Yiddish song *Ofen Pripitchik,* a song about teaching children their ABCs, quite appropriate given Bernice's career as a teacher. You can see the name of the song in the painting *Alef-Beys.* She used to be a pianist as well and often played piano in various elder communities as a volunteer. She was active as a volunteer well into her 90s.

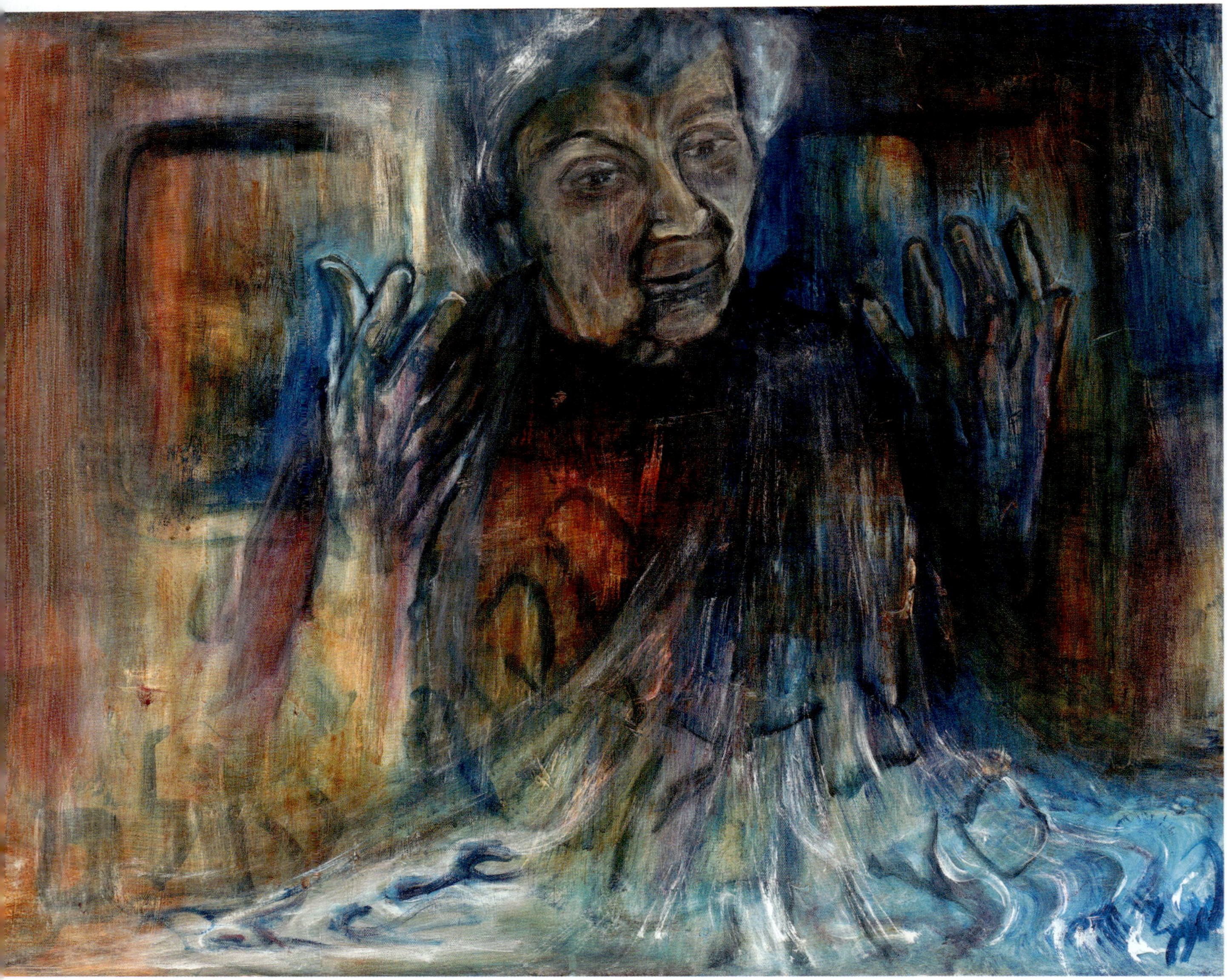

Yiddishkeit, from the story of Fannie Schanfield

Fannie Schanfield

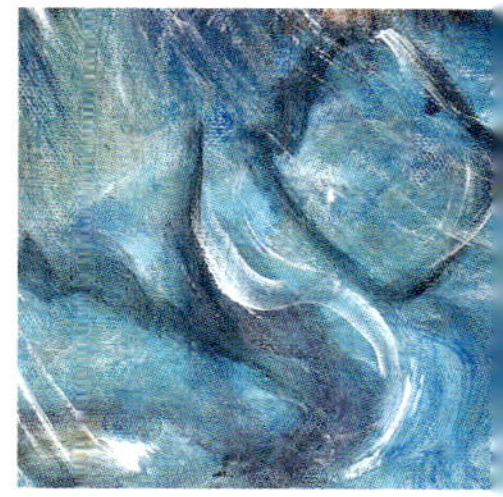

Yiddishkeit

Fannie Schanfield had once been the President of the Minneapolis chapter of *Hadassah*,[4] and I could easily imagine her successfully leading in that role. She retained a dynamic presence, expressing herself with forcefulness. Her somewhat elfin appearance belied a woman who was used to being in charge.

Those who, like Fannie, grew up surrounded by a Jewish community, did not have to think about being Jewish. It was deeply woven into the way they lived, the stores where they shopped, the language they spoke, and the neighbors who surrounded them. Still, there was an awareness of the outside community, and this awareness sometimes constrained behavior.

Fannie remembered being told not to use her hands when talking, to walk in a certain way, and to express herself in a more subdued manner. She gave a colorful explanation and defense of Yiddishkeit and the importance of it in the life of a Jew:

> *Because if you're Jewish and you don't display or tell or show that you are Jewish, you've lost it, and then we've lost it, we've lost something . . . I don't like people who are ashamed of being Jewish . . . Don't act like that, act nice, act normal.*

"So what's acting 'like that'?"

> *Well you see, you don't flip an accent, and you don't say a joke, and you don't say a Jewish word; you don't say 'Oyyyyy.' You don't use expressions like that . . . You walk straight, you don't wiggle around, and you don't sort of show so that they know you're Yiddish . . . I would use my hands. I still do today. I use my hands. . . .*
>
> *It's everything, it's everyday. Yiddishkeit is everyday. You can't just put it aside before Rosh Hashanah and Yom Kippur. Yiddishkeit has to be—so maybe you don't keep kosher—the meat is separate from the dairy,* milchig *and* fleishig*—but you maybe use the words milchig and fleishig. Maybe the* bubbe *comes home and visits and you let out a Jewish word. That's Yiddishkeit. Yiddishkeit has to be spontaneous. It isn't locked in little cubby holes . . . It's a way of living . . .*
>
> *It's part of being part of the synagogue, no matter which one it is. It's part of being, body and soul, of everyday living and believing, of what they do and knowing what it is* tzedakah *and* mitzvah*. Those are natural words and natural things, they are things that happen and you make them happen and you learn to give from the time you're that high* [she gestures] *. . . It just comes naturally, and it has to, and that's Yiddishkeit!*

How does one paint Yiddishkeit? Yiddishkeit is spontaneity, so I conjured up a waterfall of words, spilling forth with unbridled energy. If you look closely, you will see mitzvah, tzedakah, and tikkun olam. Fannie had talked about using her hands, another expression of spontaneity, so I added them. They looked rather disembodied without her face, so the rest of Fannie soon stepped in as well. Only when the painting was nearly complete did I notice that the "waterfall of words" resembled a prayer shawl, so I finished by wrapping it around her.

A Legacy of Storytelling

My theme was legacy. Unless one has acquired fame, legacy is often a subtle, quiet thing; I was to learn that story is the most important legacy of many people. A lot can be packed into a story. A story tells us of values, of family history and traditions. It tells us where we came from and the personalities of the family members who came before us.

Fannie Schanfield was a talented storyteller and recorded many of her stories in books that are held at the Berman Upper Midwest Jewish Archives. How does one become a storyteller? Fannie understood the importance of storytelling because her mother appointed Fannie, at a young age, as her spokesperson.

> *My mother was always afraid that we wouldn't remember anything she said or did, and she wanted everybody—she had six children—and she wanted the children to know that she had a life. She was a vivacious person . . . Where did she come from, what did she do and all the things that she did and saw and heard, and she was afraid it would all be forgotten. And so, she chose me as her spokesperson.*
>
> *She would always grab me in from play, and there would be a cup of coffee and milk and a caramel roll, and she'd say:* 'Es shoyn, es—*Eat, listen to what I say, and then* shrayb es arop—*write it down.*'
>
> *I said, 'uh huh, uh huh,' and I'd go be busy eating my caramel roll and drinking my coffee, and she'd keep me for about an hour, and when she was all through talking, she'd say, 'Go out to play.'*
>
> *Well, I didn't shrayb es arop. I didn't write it down.*
>
> *And one day I came home—she was staying with us—and she was burning all kinds of papers, citizenship papers, a whole bunch of them . . . on the floor in a bag. And she was destroying them.*
>
> *And I yelled, 'What are you doing?'*

> *And she says, 'Did you* shrayb, *write it down?' . . .*
>
> *At first I didn't know what she was talking about, and I said, 'No.'*
>
> *'Well, so what do I need all this for? Who's going to care? No one's going to care!'*
>
> *And then I said, 'Mama, please.'*
>
> *Well . . . she stopped destroying, and in her old age what was left my brother took, and in my old age I discovered I could write. I didn't know how, but the kids bought me a word processor. I was seventy-seven, and I remembered shrayb es arop. That would be the title . . .* Ma, I Wrote It Down.

Many of Fannie's stories revolved around artifacts that had been handed down. A multi-generational legacy began with Fannie's father, Simon Schwartz, who was a *chazan* at B'nai Emet. Fannie told us:

> *In 1926 or '27, I don't recall exactly, there was a fire in the* shtiebel, *attached to the synagogue on 13th Avenue and 9th Street. And he* [her father] *was quite discouraged, and he thought that there should be electric lights. They ought to have lamps with electricity in them so they could move them and not cause fires like this. And he thought about it, and he thought about it, and one day he was walking home from synagogue with his neighbor, and he was discussing the situation, how bad it is, and he, Mr. Osias Silvers, said he was a smith, works with materials and makes things, a tinsmith, and he thinks he could make a reasonable pair of candlesticks.*
>
> *So, Pa said, 'You mean if I get you drawings and patterns, you will be able to make an actual thing?'*
>
> *'Oh sure,' he said. He does that every day for a living.*
>
> *And so, they started. Mr. Silvers went back to work, and he asked his boss if he could have some metal strips, scraps that they didn't want to use anymore, so that he could make something for the synagogue. The guy says, 'Sure,' so along the floor he picked up some brass strips and some metal . . . And he put them in a bag and in a box, and he brought them home. And he said, 'Mr. Schwartz,'—nobody called anyone by their first name—'Mr. Schwartz, could you make something out of these strips of scraps?'*
>
> *And he said, 'You know, I think we can make some candlesticks.' Okay, so he put them away, and Pa went to work and designed a pair of candelabras . . . They're over five feet tall, and he specified to be electrified for electricity. And he brought them to Mr. Silvers, and he said if we had a drawing he could cut it out. He has instruments and things that could cut the metal . . . just like a pattern on a dress.*
>
> *So, Papa set about getting paper long enough, and he had someone help him draw the outline of what he wanted, and it was made. The patterns were made, and he brought them to Mr. Silvers and said, 'Could you work from this?' Absolutely he could*

work from this with a few exceptions, and they set about making the patterning for the candelabras. And they came to be . . . with these two colors of metal . . . And you can go to the synagogue and see.

Years later, after B'nai Emet moved to St. Louis Park in the 1950s, Fannie went in search of the candelabras. Finding them in ill repair, she paid to have them refurbished. Ultimately, they stood at her daughter's wedding, carrying her father's legacy forward to one more generation.

I asked Fannie if she had something from the past that was still part of her life today, and she answered without hesitation:

> Benching licht, *benching licht—blessing the candles on Friday night. My grandmother, who came to live with us, had her set of candles; my mother had her set of candles. And you see when my mother, when they were packing her up to ship her to America so she could marry her boyfriend, you see the first thing that his mother put in the trunk was a pair of candlesticks. They are over 200 years old.*

She walked over to her dining room and pointed out the candlesticks that had made the journey in her mother's trunk.

All of Fannie's stories related to fire, light, and legacy, so that became the name of the painting. As I thought of these stories filled with light, I decided to make the background the color of fire. Many of Fannie's stories included legacy in a tangible form, be it candelabras or Sabbath candlesticks. I began to pull out the suggestion of the candelabras in the background and incorporated an image I had of her mother as the central figure holding the flaming papers of her legacy. A candle in the 200-year-old candlestick symbolizes the passing of time.

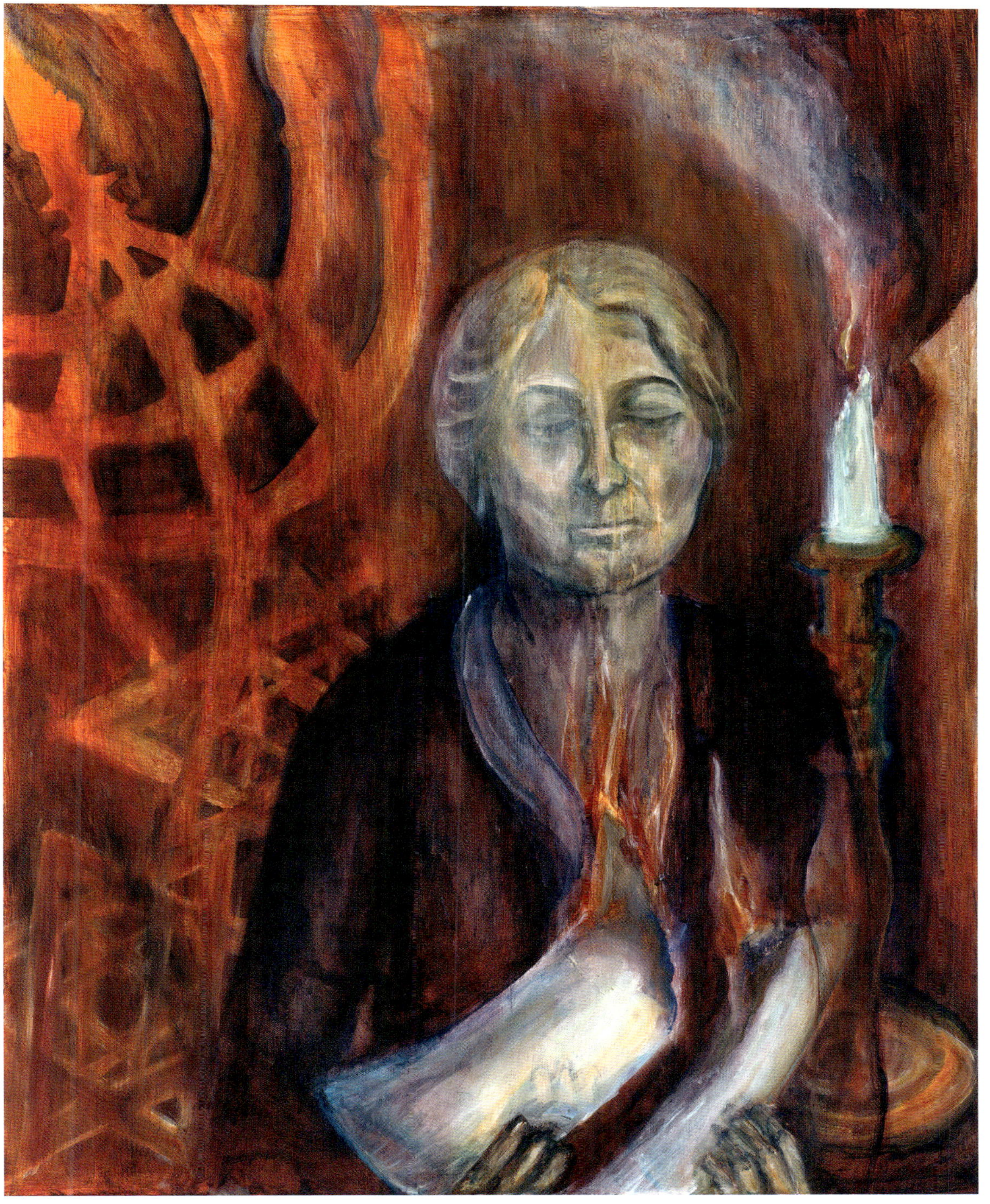

Fire, Light, and Legacy, from the story of Fannie Schanfield

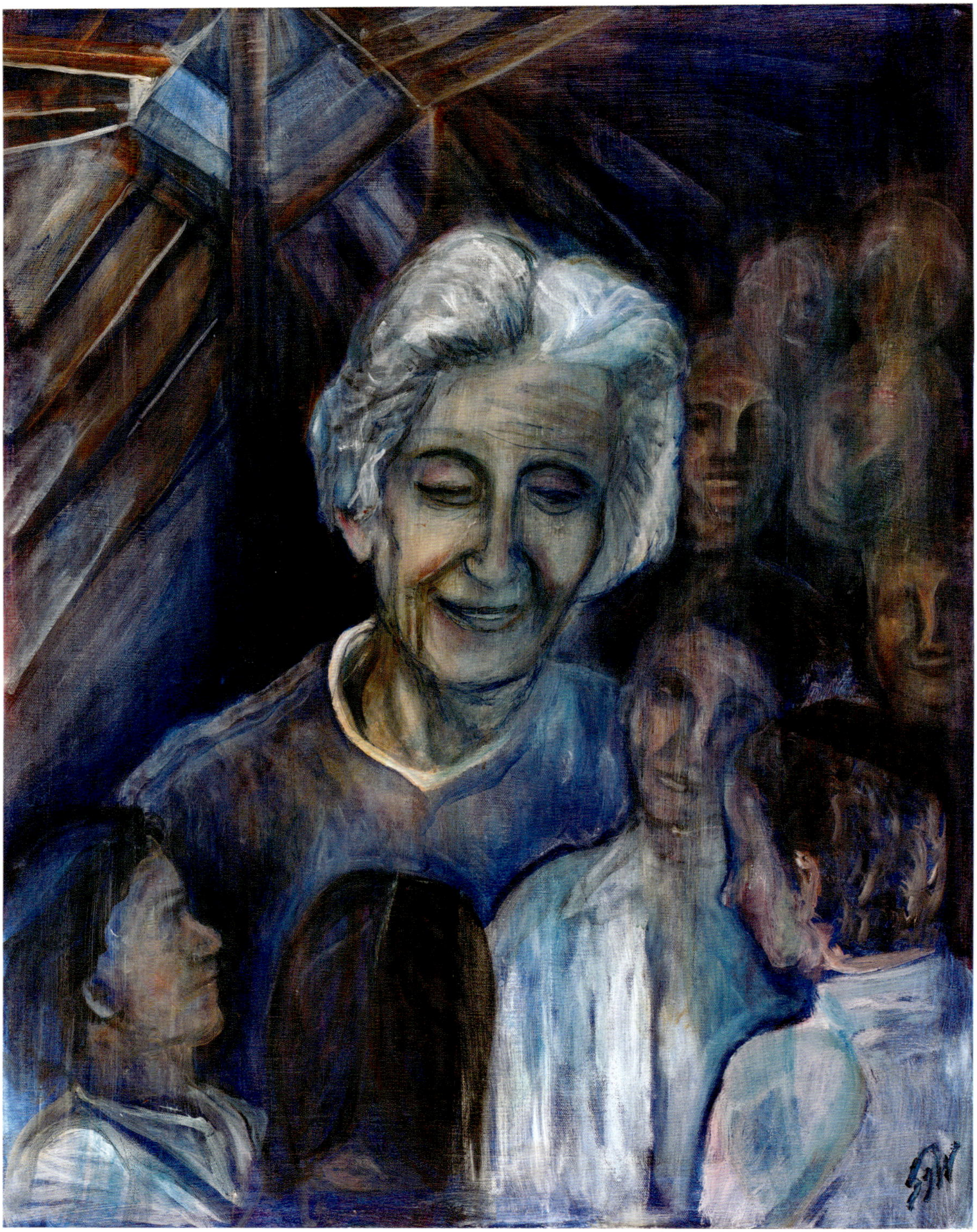

Grandma Zelda, from the story of Zelda Katz

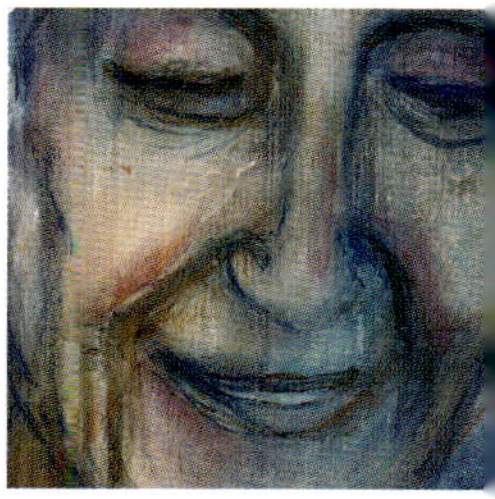

Zelda Katz

A Legacy of Relationship

Zelda Katz had a long face topped with white hair washed with grey. Her voice was gruff, a bit husky. For Zelda, legacy took the form of relationships, especially those with children. Known as "Grandma Zelda" to the Beth Jacob congregation, she was adopted by many of the children, and in turn by their families. Zelda Katz grew up on St. Paul's West Side. She worked with children at Children's Hospital as a nursing assistant for more than 40 years. "I was glad when they went home, the little darlings, and I would tell them, 'Don't come back, we don't have no Disneyland here'."

When we asked her how she came to wear the honorific of Grandma Zelda, she told this story:

I always loved children, and they know it. The kids at Beth Jacob know it. I'm only known as Grandma Zelda, Grandma Zelda. Two little boys came up to me, and one said, 'Hi, Grandma Zelda. How are you?'

And the other one looked at him and said, 'She your grandma?'

And the first one said, 'Yes, she's my grandma, and she's everybody's grandma.' And he goes like this [pointing] *'And listen, she could be your grandma, too, if you want her to.'*

So the second one said, 'Do you think she would be?'

And the first one said, 'All you have to do is ask her.'

So he comes up to me, and he says, 'Can I ask you something?'

And I kiddingly said, 'Is it going to cost me money?'

And he said, 'No . . . Would you be my Grandma Zelda?'

I almost—I had tears in my eyes. I says, 'I would be happy to be your Grandma Zelda, but when you see me, what are you going to say to me?'

'No problem, if it's on Shabbos, I'll say: Good Shabbos, Grandma Zelda. If it's on any other time, I'll say: Hi, Grandma Zelda. How are you?'

Kids to me are beautiful. I love children. I'll take all the time in the world to talk to them, and if they have anything to say that they want me to help them, I'll be there for them. 'Cause I love kids.

I was never married, [she added in a gravelly voice] *but I have a lot of grandchildren.*

Zelda was an important person at Beth Jacob, where everyone had a Grandma Zelda story to share. When I painted her story, I knew she had to be a central presence surrounded by children. An architectural feature of Beth Jacob can be found at the top, representing the location for these relationships. I had the opportunity to observe first-hand how closely identified Zelda was with her title of Grandma Zelda. When some visitors to my studio saw the painting, one exclaimed, "It's Grandma Zelda!"

Anne Milavetz

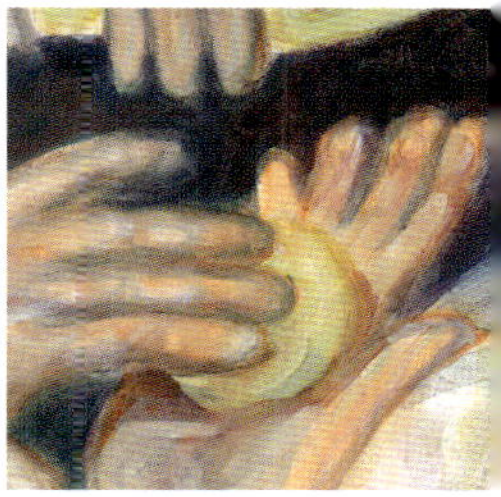

Sharing Traditions

Most of our interviews were with elders who had lived in the Twin Cities. When we met with Anne Milavetz, we heard a very different experience. Anne was born in Winnipeg, but lived in Virginia, Minnesota after her marriage. Virginia is part of the Iron Range, an area in Northern Minnesota where Jewish communities have largely disappeared Anne had fond memories of this community. Today the area has a population of about 9,000 and, according to her report, only two remaining Jews.

Anne's was a gentle presence. A cloud of white hair formed soft waves around her face. She wore a pale pink sweater, and pearl earrings caught the light as she turned toward us. We met in her Sholom apartment where a photograph of a man standing in the glow of a stained-glass window quickly drew our attention. Anne explained that the photo was of her late husband, Daniel, taken in B'nai Abraham, their synagogue in Virginia. She reported the survival of that synagogue with pride, despite the loss of the Jewish community it once served.

> *This is the only city in the area of the Iron Range, in the Jewish community, that . . . survived with our synagogue . . . we all donated, and it now belongs to the city of Virginia, and they can use it for . . . things like music . . . He* [her husband] *would have been so thrilled. Because he loved that synagogue . . .*
>
> *Most of the synagogues on the Range were destroyed or made churches. They didn't want to do that to this synagogue because it really was a beautiful synagogue.*

Anne had warm memories of the community of Virginia, where she opened her home to her friends and neighbors. She fondly remembered her life there, but it was a memory tinged with sadness since the community had dispersed.

> *Our house was open, and they'd bring their kids in buggies and baskets, and that's what we wanted. We wanted our house open to the people we loved. But, you know, it's a sad story when they're all gone . . .*
>
> *We had a wonderful time at holidays . . . I had a big house, and I liked company. I had a lot of people who didn't have places to go. They would come to my house. We had our little synagogue which we all loved. We had a pretty good group of young people. But you see what happened is we all got older and left, and there are* [only] *two people left . . .*

I really liked living [there]. *We had a* Hadassah. *We had every organization the Jewish people have in the cities, on a smaller scale, and we made different affairs to raise money. It was wonderful living there . . .*

I think we had about forty [Jewish] *families . . . Never had a rabbi. We always had these roving rabbis. But we always had men in the town who were very well-versed who could do a service . . .*

We went to Duluth [for kosher food]. *And I had a big freezer upstairs and a big freezer downstairs because I kept kosher, because I wanted my in-laws to come and eat with me.*

While others in these interviews spoke of antisemitism in housing or alluded to it in finding employment, Anne fondly remembered sharing traditions with her non-Jewish neighbors. In a small town where there was more opportunity for interaction, she felt very much a part of the community. Unlike the experience several noted in the Twin Cities, Anne expressed that she did not experience antisemitism on the Iron Range of Northern Minnesota.

I never once met a person that I thought was antisemitic. My friends in Virginia, [some] *were . . . Gentiles. And they had us for Christmas, and I had them for Yom Kippur . . . They learned how to make knishes. I taught them how to make knishes. I used to make bagels. We were the best of friends. I never knew anything like . . .* [antisemitism] *there.*

In deciding how to capture this in paint, I decided to paint the sharing of traditions. I studied videos of people making knishes and combined them in an image of hands engaged in a shared activity. Behind them is the suggestion of a Christmas tree to reflect the sharing of traditions.

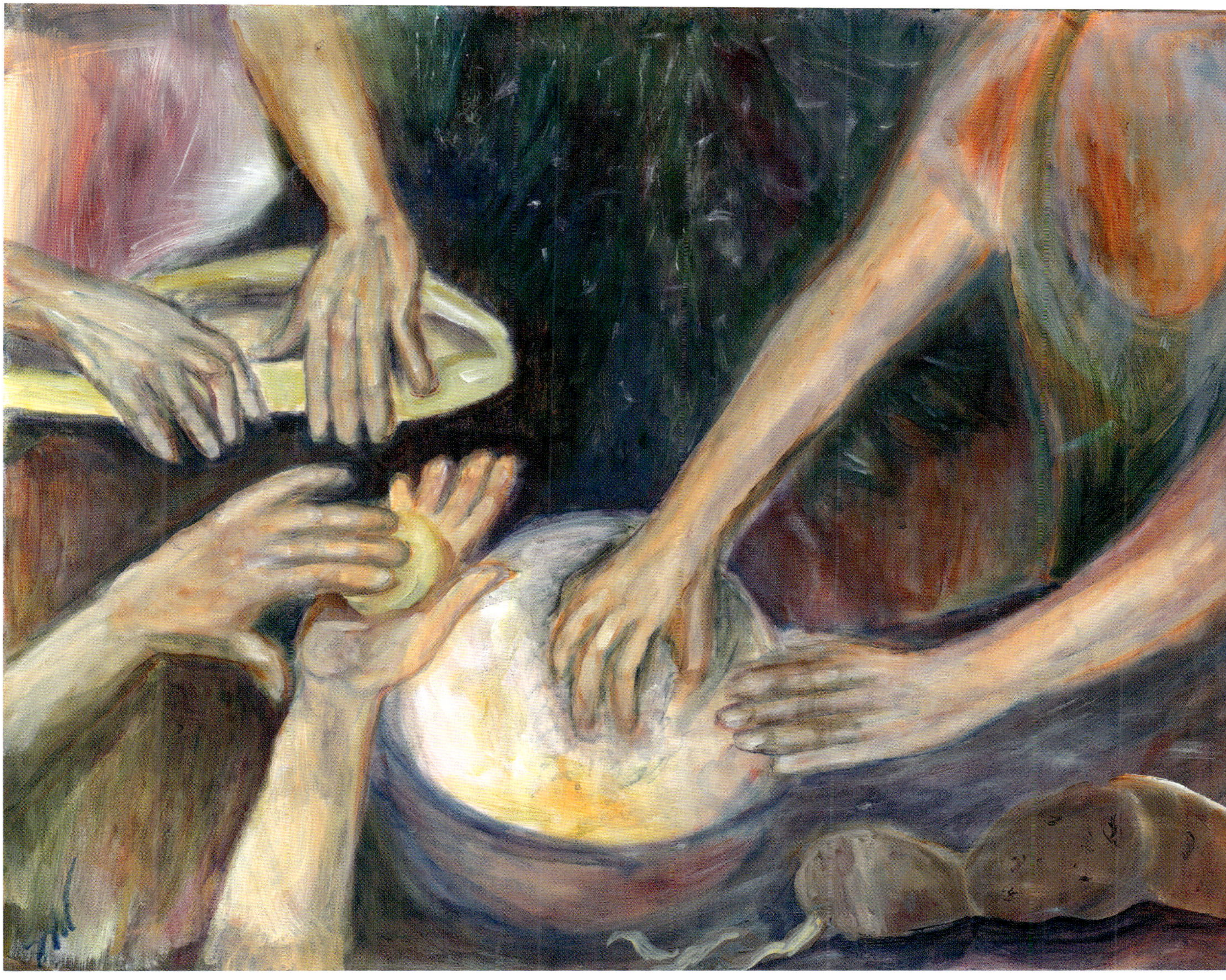

Making Knishes, from the story of Anne Milavetz

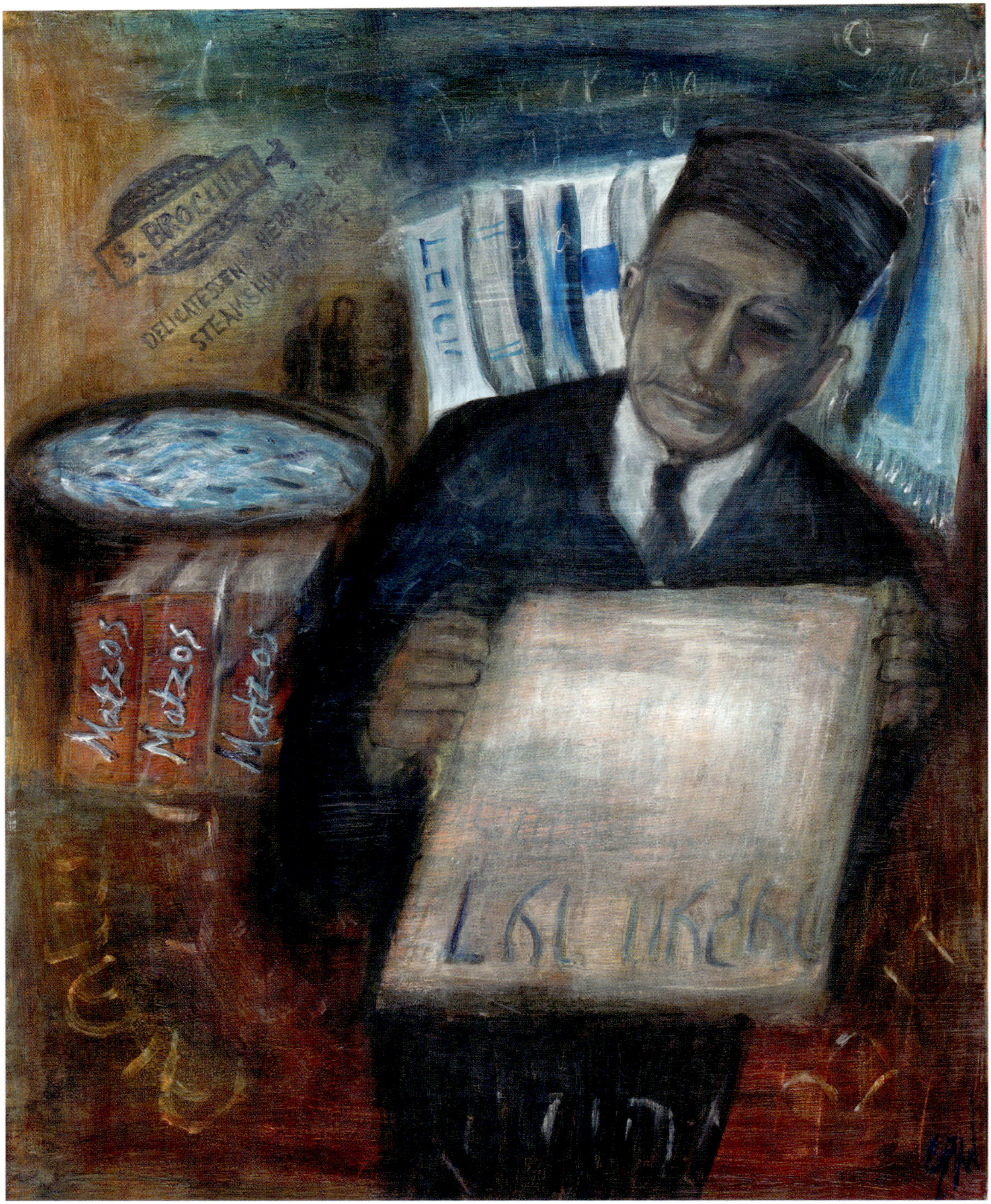

Body and Soul, from the story of Dorothy Brochin Wittcoff

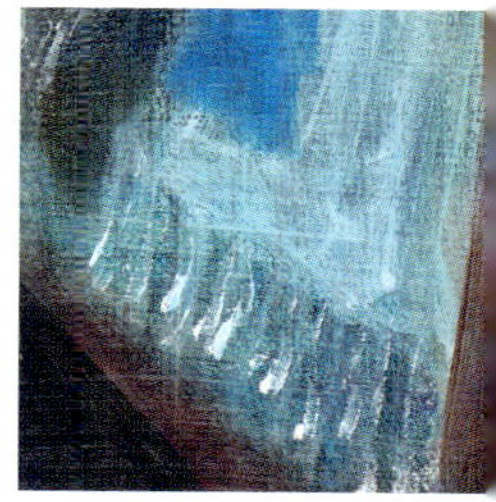

Dorothy Brochin Wittcoff

Body and Soul

Dorothy Brochin Wittcoff was tiny and soft-spoken, with a delicate frame. As her story unfolded, I began to understand both her deep roots in her family and her spirit of adventure. There was a large presence in that small frame. Dorothy sat beside her husband, Harold, and their son and granddaughter joined us.

Dorothy's parents, Solomon and Anna Brochin, having decided they were not going to raise their family under the threat of pogroms, arrived in Minneapolis in 1906. By 1909, Solomon Brochin was listed in the city directory as a Minneapolis confectioner.[5] His grocery store soon became a fixture on the North Side. In addition to its offerings of corned beef and Yiddish newspapers, the store served as a community center for the Jewish neighborhood.

> *My father was one of the founders of the Jewish community here . . . and he had the first kosher grocery store, which took up half of the store, and the other half was devoted to Jewish books and* taleisim *and things of that type because there was absolutely nobody who was taking care of that particular need.*

Dorothy remembered when Louis Brandeis was touring Jewish communities around 1916 and came to the Brochins' store. Chaim Weitzman also visited.

> *We were little kids, but my father said to us, 'You should go and say hello because these* [people] *are going to be hugely important to the Jewish community.'*

She described the family of her childhood.

> *He had seven children, and I was number five . . . Isadore, Ben, Ida, Adele, Dorothy, Joe, and then comes Gloria . . . My mother worked in the store right with him . . .*

Dorothy told how the children all received their American names at school.

> *All of us got our English names from the kindergarten teacher at school . . . like my Hebrew name was Dvora, and it began with a D, and I became Dorothy I don't know how Adele got her name. Her name was Judith. Ida . . . was Shoshana, and Ben was Benyamin.*

With her son, Ralph, Dorothy traced one brother's name from the original She'ar Yashuv, which was shortened to Yashu, which was shorted to Osh, and eventually became Joe.

She continued, "Then, of course, my younger sister was Galooya, which means 'freedom.'"

"Which became Gloria," said Ralph.

Dorothy married a young man whom she had known as a child. He was killed as an aviator in World War II, a month before Ralph was born. Three years later she remarried.

Helping Those in Need

> *I was a young widow at that time. They—members of the Jewish community—decided we would be a good match, so from two different sources, he was told that maybe he ought to go see [me].*

Two years after their marriage, Dorothy and her husband, Harold, added Mike, a foster child, to their family. And later came Ted, their third son.

> *We have a foster child that I took in who came out of the camps. And I took him in on a temporary basis. I was with a Jewish agency at the time. We got a note from New York: 'We're sending you ten boys. Find homes. You can place them temporarily, but we have to get them out of New York. They just came out of the* DP [Displaced Persons] *camps.'*
>
> *So I said, 'I'll take one, temporary.' So I took Mike, and he came to live in our house.*

"Temporary" was quickly forgotten. Mike became a permanent family member. Ralph was five at the time and immediately viewed ten-year-old Mike as his older brother. Ralph noted:

> *At the age of ten,* [Mike] *was in the underground, smuggling people and weapons in and out of the camps. He was the guy who was passing as a Polish peasant lad on the haystack, with partisans buried underneath.*

An Adventurous Life

Dorothy shared a life of adventure with Harold. She became a medical social worker, and later she also taught English, while accompanying her husband around the world on his travels for consulting work. Dorothy was especially enthusiastic when she spoke about teaching in China, shortly after it opened to foreign visitors.

> *I taught in China; that was one of the most interesting groups I had . . . I taught them English . . . I did a survey on the class to find out how many different levels there were. Then I went down to . . . where they had books for sale and did quite a survey of what was available. And then I took some back to the classroom . . . We looked all through these books, and they decided which ones they felt they could benefit from . . . They were so tremendously eager to learn, and they would learn ahead before I was even there. That was a tremendous experience.*

Perhaps her son, Ralph, described her best:

> *When she saw a need, she did something about it . . . For a diminutive person, she could be very forceful.*[6]

When I turned to painting, I was struck by the importance of Dorothy's family history. Her roots ran deeply into the fabric of the Jewish community. Her family was proud of their history, and their stories had been oft-told. I decided to focus on those roots through a painting of Solomon Brochin, Dorothy's father, holding a Yiddish newspaper in his store. I wanted the painting to show that one side of the store sold groceries, while the other was for religious articles, and Jewish books and newspapers.

After I had completed the painting, I was visited by Dorothy and Ralph at my studio. She stood before the painting, studying it as she gripped her walker with Ralph by her side. I nervously awaited the verdict. She confirmed that it looked like him, but there was an adjustment required: he wasn't wearing a *yarmulke,* and he had always worn one at the store. Conveniently, I had a collage with a photo of my own great-grandfather wearing a square yarmulke. She nodded, "Yes, like that." Of course, I painted one like it for Dorothy's father.

The story of the kindergarten naming ritual, when Hebrew names were discarded for Americanized versions, is also reflected in this painting. I included the names in Hebrew at the bottom, while their Americanized versions are at the top. Since this painting is based on Dorothy's story, you can also find her Hebrew name—*Dvora*—on one of the *tallitot* behind her father.

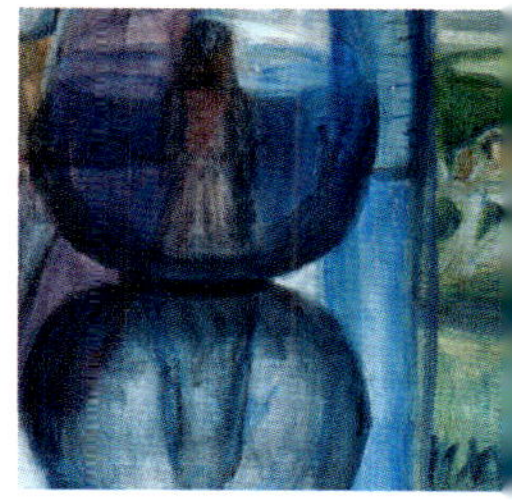

Harold Wittcoff

The Second Jew

Harold Wittcoff sat beside his wife, Dorothy, during our interview and reached out to take her hand into his. Their relationship was clearly an important part of their story, one with many elements of *beshert*. He recalled a recent walk into shul when they had met the rabbi:

> *We were talking . . . and I said something very nice happened to us. It was our 66th wedding anniversary this week. So, he gave us an* aliyah.

Harold was a soft-spoken man and an enthusiastic storyteller. He had accomplished much in his life, but he made a point of drawing out Dorothy's story as well. I was touched by them, both by the natural affection they evidenced as a couple and by the high regard and respect he clearly held for her accomplishments.

Dorothy was a war widow with a young toddler when she met Harold. Their paths kept crossing, with a little assistance from community members who had rightly decided they would be good together. In 1946 the Wittcoffs married, and together they raised their family in Minneapolis. When Harold retired after 35 years, Dorothy left her job as the director of social work at a local hospital. Then, together, they traveled the world.

After retirement, Harold worked with a consulting firm where he developed and taught a course on industrial chemistry. While he taught chemistry, Dorothy taught English. They lived in Israel, London, and New York and taught in places as far flung as Southeast Asia, Japan, Africa, and South America. Harold didn't retire for the second time until he was 91. This was a couple who were clearly well matched, and they thrived on an adventurous life.

Harold was not a native Minnesotan. He was raised by immigrant parents in Marion, Indiana, an area he reported was not a good place to be Jewish:

> *The Ku Klux Klan had an office right next to my father's tailor shop. And so they would have parades on Washington Street in their sheets and headdresses . . . So, there was a tremendous amount of antisemitism.*

Harold came to Minneapolis in the 1940s, a time coinciding with Minneapolis being labeled "the capitol [*sic*] of antisemitism in the United States" by writer Carey McWilliams.[7]

Harold moved to Minneapolis to work for a large food company. He had just finished his PhD at Northwestern, and the company made him a job offer, something that Harold noted was not the norm in those times:

> *It was not so easy for Jewish boys to get offers, but it got easier all of a sudden, because this is during the war . . . 1943, and the government is . . . giving money to companies who start research operations. So, all these companies wanted to start research operations, and they needed researchers, so all the graduates had no trouble getting jobs. . . .*
>
> *I was the second Jew to get a job at* [this company] *by the way. The first was Mr. Goldberg, who was the janitor. I became, in the end, Vice President . . . and as far as I know that's unique. I don't know of any other* [Jewish] *vice presidents* [there].

When I turned to painting, I thought about my reaction to our interview. I was struck by the Wittcoffs' loving relationship and the spirit of adventure they shared, traversing the world together with Harold teaching chemistry and Dorothy teaching English. The image of Harold putting his hand over Dorothy's stayed with me, seeming to capture the spirit of their marriage. In the painting, this gentle embrace forms a shelter resting upon the world of their travels.

I decided to use chemistry as a motif, as that was both Harold's professional expertise and reflective of his relationship with his wife. Within each flask, you will find elements of their story, along with a shadow beneath to represent underlying memory. Memories are, in fact, shadows of actual events, impressions that stay with us. Dorothy's first husband died in WWII, leaving her a young widow with a child when she met Harold. Ralph told a story of the return from their wedding, when Harold first said he was Ralph's new daddy. I decided to make the color of this vial red, representing the binding strength of these new family connections.

A blue vial represents a gateway to the ocean voyage of Harold's mother. He had described her immigration to the United States and her wonder at the glass ceiling of the Hamburg train station:

> *She got to Hamburg, and she used to say that the most remarkable thing that she saw was the railroad station that had a glass ceiling. And she'd say, 'Of course it isn't there anymore, but it was a remarkable thing to see.' Well, I was in Hamburg, and I went to the railroad station and, sure enough, it has a glass ceiling.*

The Wittcoffs were very involved with Labor Zionism, and their son remembers they went to gatherings when he was a child where people dressed in white and did Israeli dances. You can see the memory of those dancers within the green beaker.

The chemical structures of salt and sugar are suggested in the lower left and upper right. Both flavorful crystals symbolize a satisfying life.

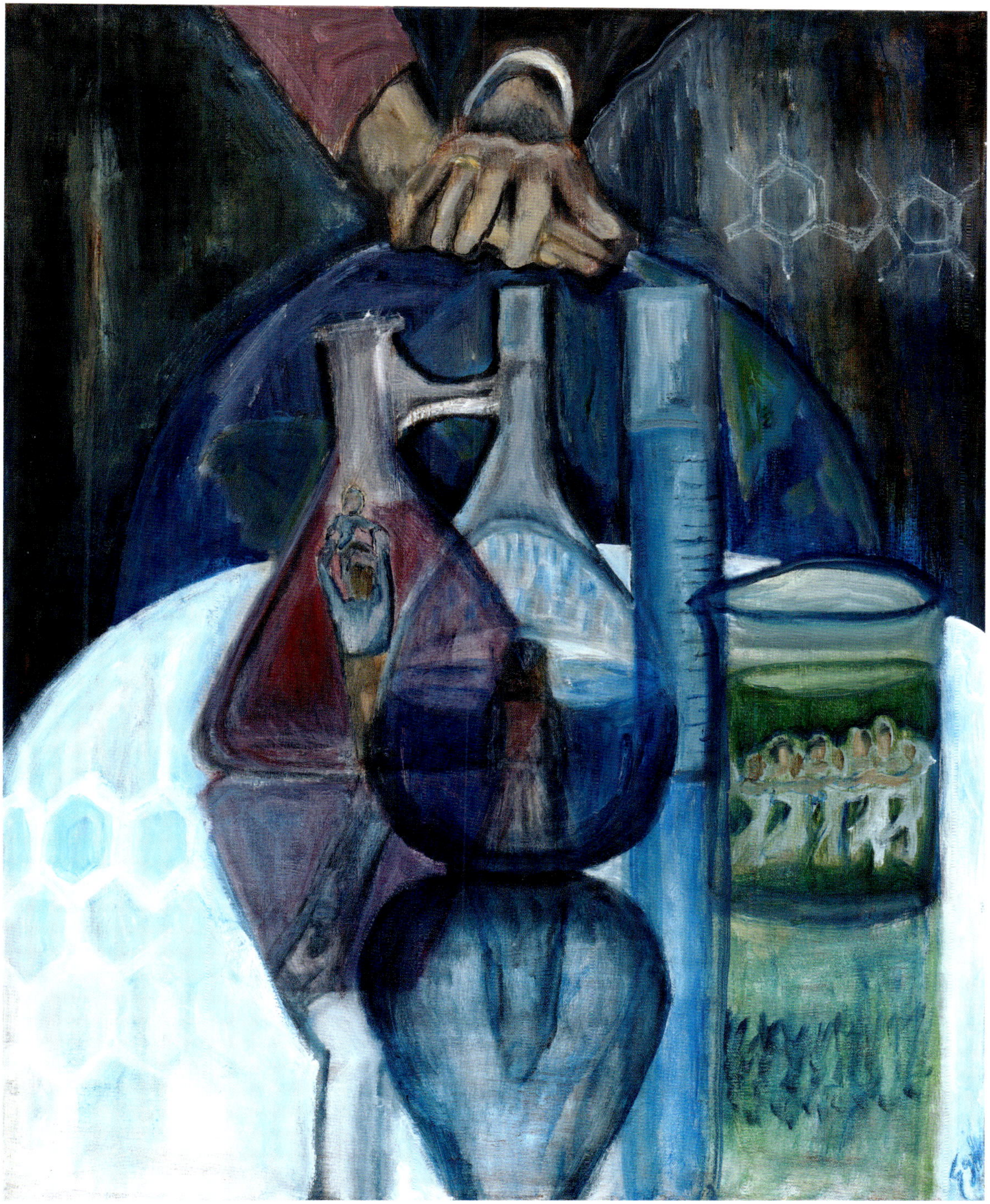

A Matter of Chemistry, from the story of Harold Wittcoff

A Few Thoughts

The children of the early immigrants grew up with one foot in each world. Jewish immigrants were their neighbors as well as their family. Customs were carried over from European roots, as Shirley learned at her grandmother's bedside, where she was greeted by tomorrow's dinner. Children spoke Jewish at home and in their community. School was the point of demarcation where they entered the broader world, the English-speaking world.

To the extent that they were ensconced in the Jewish community, this group was often protected from the antisemitism that lurked on their doorstep. That antisemitism might urge them to fit in and not appear too outwardly Jewish, a pressure that Fannie rejected with a full-throated appeal to Yiddishkeit. In small-town Minnesota, Anne had a very different experience. Finding all the Jewish organizations scaled down to size and a welcoming (rather than antisemitic) community, Anne welcomed others to her home and took pleasure in many warm relationships. Her later experience reflects the dwindling presence of Jews in these towns as young people were attracted to more urban areas.

Each individual claimed their place: Shirley as an exuberant storyteller, Anne as a warm hostess, Zelda as every child's warm-hearted *bubbe,* Fannie as a leader in Hadassah and a writer of stories, and Bernice as an educator and talented musician. Dorothy and Harold demonstrated the emergence of highly-educated community leaders who offered their talents in the broader world, while still holding deep ties to their heritage.

Of Loss and Survival

Holocaust survivors shared stories of losing both family and community. Some were trapped in Europe during the war, surviving concentration camps and forced labor. Even those who escaped Europe on the cusp of the war lost family members. Some came to the United States in the mid-1940s and early 1950s. Many remained in Germany after the war, a main location of DP camps, while awaiting an opportunity to leave. It was not until immigration laws changed that access to the United States became more available.

Upon immigrating, their story shifts to one of reconstructing life in a new country: learning a language, training for a career, and building new family connections and friendships. Each of them married and began a family, focusing on their new future in the United States.

The Holocaust stories all have similar elements of loss and disruption, but each is also quite unique, defined by the drama of personal stories. Each is a story of a journey, and many of the paintings are collage-like to capture the complexity of these stories.

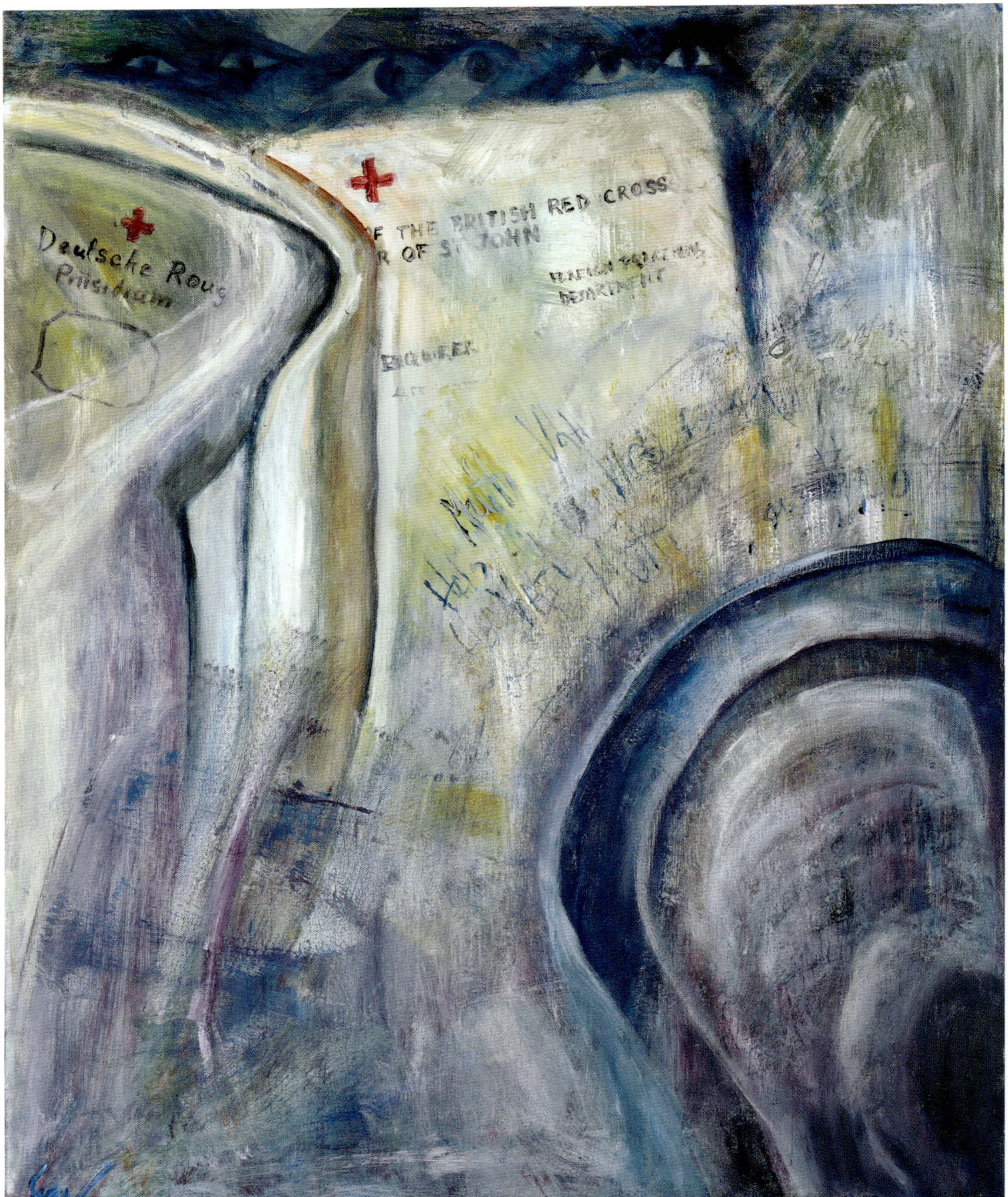

Everything Stopped, from the story of Hanna Lyon

Hanna Lyon

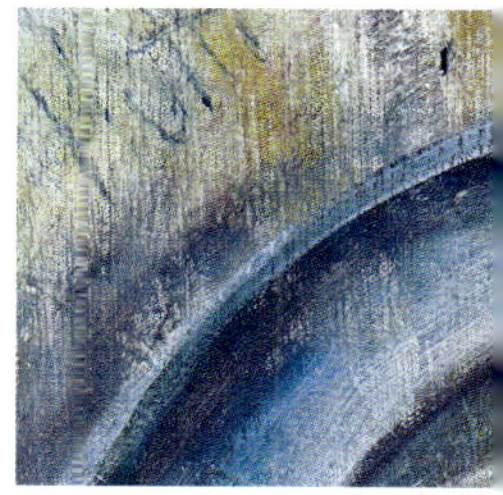

The Kindertransport

We met with Hanna Lyon in her apartment at Sholom. Her two daughters and two granddaughters joined us. They noted that they knew pieces of Hanna's story but were curious to see if more would emerge.

Hanna had a close-cropped cap of white hair and a slight German accent. She sat on the couch surrounded by family members with picture albums piled at her feet. She began by commenting on how she didn't talk about the Holocaust. "I never bothered the children with the Holocaust and all that. I never told them anything."

Hanna had arrived in Minnesota after living in England, where she had been sent as part of the *Kindertransport*. This was a rescue effort focused on bringing children from Germany and German-occupied territories out to safety. From 1938–39, approximately 10,000 children were sent to foster homes in England. Many became the only survivors from their families. Hanna had lived a comfortable life in Germany. When she left for England, she learned to speak the language and acclimated to a different life. Her experience was deeply touched by loneliness and loss, as her parents and brother remained behind and ultimately died in Auschwitz:

> *When I was sixteen, I emigrated to England. I was all on my own already. My mother packed my suitcase and whatever she wanted me to take to America later on. I went to England with the children's transport. I went to a very nice family who needed help for their kids and taking care of the house. A Quaker family. I went to church with them on Sunday, a different life.*
>
> *I got Red Cross letters from my parents. They were still alive at that time, but how much longer nobody knows. I never talked to them since Germany, since I left . . .*
>
> *You didn't write much because you knew somebody else was in between . . .*
>
> *I was very lonesome, the only person having to go from my house. Lots of other kids went, too, and different ages. For me it was awful . . . I had everything at home. I never had to do anything. Then, all of a sudden, you work, and the English people are very fussy. The bricks in front of the fireplaces—they have polished bricks, and they had to be polished every day . . .*
>
> *I spoke French and German, but no English. I learned English with my dictionary.*

I had a German-English dictionary. I still have it. I had that with me all the time. The lady was very nice. That couple was very nice, and the child. So they taught me. You learn. When you're young, you learn easier than when you're older . . .

And then I had those Red Cross letters. I still have them . . . then everything stopped.

As we spoke Hanna held an album on her lap filled with photographs from Germany and the Red Cross letters, her last communication with her parents, lovingly preserved. Her hands moved over the letters as if to extract her parents' presence. She continued telling her story.

After three years in England, I learned I wanted to be a nurse. I started my training in England. It was during the war already because I took care of soldiers in an army hospital . . . I went into nurses' training, so I was at the nursing home or at those homes, and the rest I had my own apartment with a girlfriend. We shared that, which was freedom. I didn't finish nursing [school] *in England. There wasn't enough time. So, I finished it here, in Minneapolis . . .*

Life in America was so much different. In England, it's everything tea, and tea again. I haven't touched a glass of tea since I've been in America. It doesn't taste good anymore.

Hanna was fortunate to have an uncle in Minneapolis. He had first lived in South Africa where he learned English, before joining his then-girlfriend in Minneapolis. They became family for Hanna.

The couple was the best thing for me. They took over [for] *my parents. They made everything for me . . . He went to America because he had a girlfriend in Germany who was already in America, and she had a brother here who had a store on Nicollet Avenue, a ready-to-wear store. They got married, and they brought me over from England to America, and I stayed with them in their house, on the davenport sleeping, for six months. And then I went to finish my nursing training.*

Hanna's story was best told in what wasn't said. In answer to the question of how she knew her parents were no longer alive, she replied, "Everything stopped," and I knew that would be the name of the painting even before I began to paint. This was a painting that I started by writing poetry, as I struggled to find my way into the deep sadness. I pictured a void of silence, a black hole, and began to paint it in the corner of the canvas. As I painted the black hole, it reminded me of an ear, the dark center of it, listening anxiously for word that doesn't come. It occurred to me there must have been a long period of waiting, listening, before the finality of "everything stopped" was acknowledged. It would have been a gradual, horrifying realization. As I thought of Hanna's experience at that time, the concept of the painting began to take form. It was to be of that moment before full comprehension of loss, when one anxiously awaits the word that doesn't come, the pit-in-the-stomach kind of waiting.

The form of an ear began to take shape. Blues and purples seemed like the right colors, with blue the color of sadness, loss. Above are the scratched-in words, *Mutti, Vati* (Mother, Father) and *Halo* (their pet name for her), words that were written in the Red Cross letters. Eyes watch from the top of the painting.

After I had finished this series of paintings, I gave a talk on the project. Hanna was in the audience, and this was the first time she would see the painting. I was a bit uneasy. It wasn't a representational painting, and I didn't know how she would respond. I was pleased when she spoke with some surprise of how it captured exactly what she had felt.

For a time the paintings were at Sholom, where she lived. A friend stopped by to see the show and encountered Hanna, who shared the story behind the painting with her, giving it an added resonance. There was a sense of ownership that arose about this painting. It was her story after all.

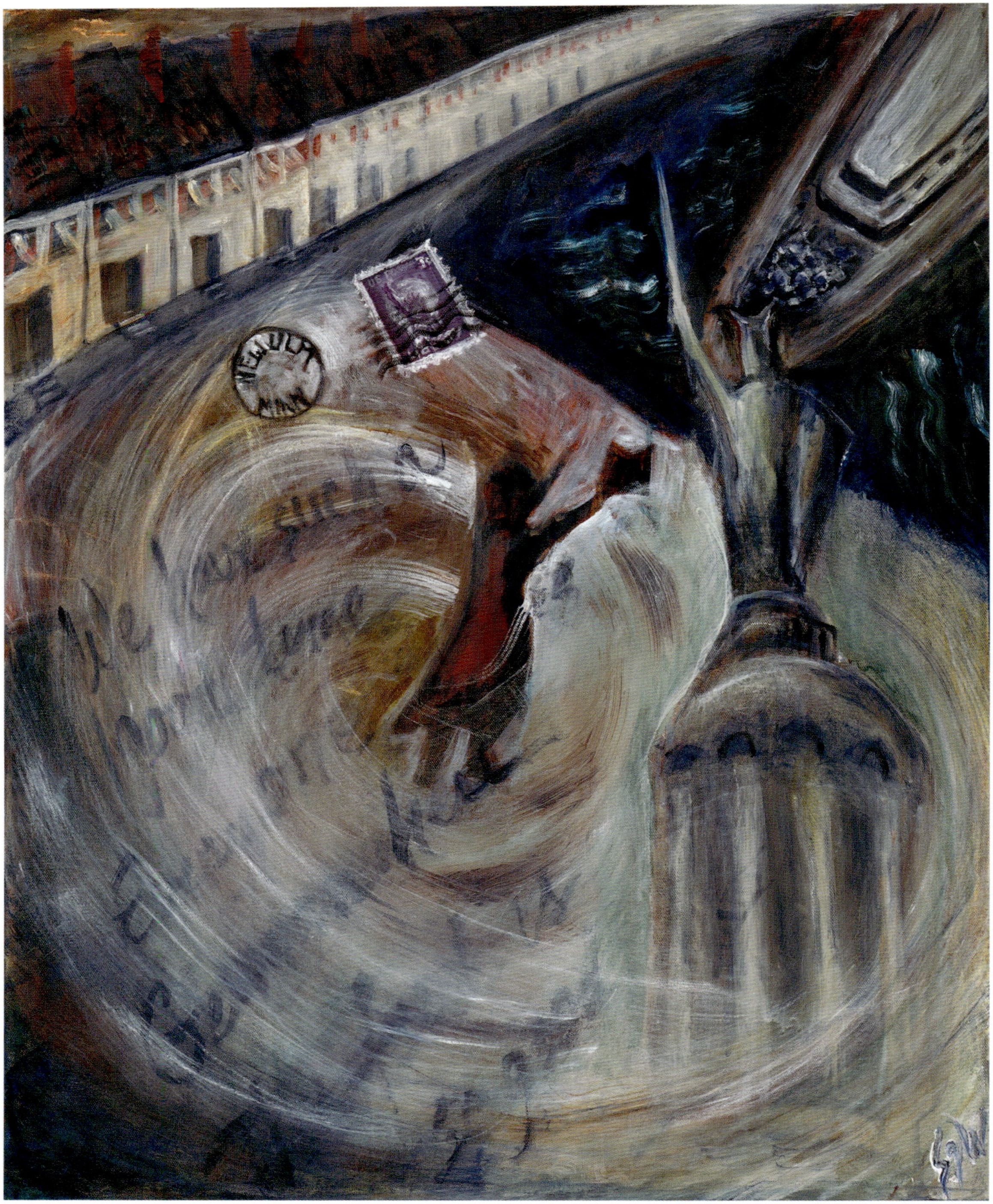

Postcard from New Ulm, from the story of Trudy Rappaport

Trudy Rappaport

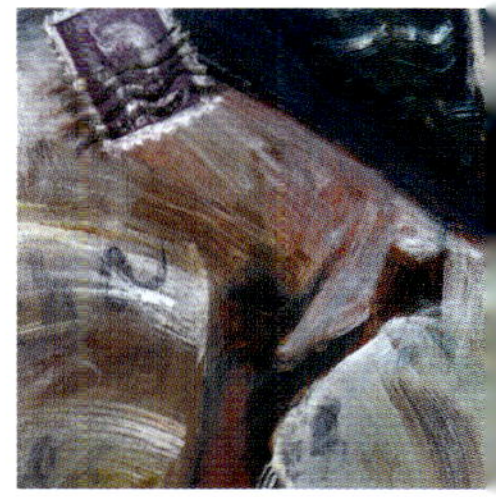

Stuck in Germany

Like Hanna Lyon, Trudy Rappaport also lived in Germany. Both young women had seen the Holocaust begin to unfold much earlier than people living elsewhere in Europe. While Poland was not invaded until 1939, Germany first saw the impact in 1933, when there was still time to escape, for those prescient enough about what was yet to come.

Trudy joined us in an activity room at the Sholom facility where she lived. Red geraniums lined the window as sunshine flooded the room. Wavy white hair framed an expressive face, and she spoke with a German accent. It was hard for her to speak of the Holocaust, but Trudy proved to be an exceptional storyteller.

"Do I have to talk about it?" she plaintively asked as she settled in across from me.

"You can tell me what you are comfortable discussing," I replied, wondering what that would leave.

In fact, with permission to stop at any point of discomfort, Trudy spoke freely about her experience. She presented the beginning of the Nazi regime through a young girl's eyes, with the loss of a friend.

> *I had a good friend, a girlfriend. She was my age, and we went to school together. We were close. She lived just around the corner from where I lived. Sometimes I stayed overnight at her house, she stayed overnight at my house. She was not Jewish. And it was about '33, all of a sudden my girlfriend was a little strange toward me.*
>
> *And one day she came and said, 'Trudy, I cannot be friends with you anymore.'*
>
> *I said, 'Why?'*
>
> *'Because my father worked for the radio station, and if they find out that I am having a Jewish friend, then he will lose his job.'*
>
> *So that was the beginning. I lost her. We couldn't get jobs anymore. I didn't go to school anymore.*

Life soon worsened as the Nazi noose tightened. Trudy was fifteen when her education ended. She finally found a job at a factory that was in Jewish hands. After a few years, they were forced to sell, and she lost her job.

Then came Kristallnacht . . . *1938. In the morning, they came and arrested my father, took him away. Didn't know where they took him. It took us quite a few days to find out. They took him to a concentration camp. Sachsenhausen, near Berlin.*

We had to move. Our landlord who was not Jewish told us we had to move, so we moved in with my uncle and aunt. They had a big apartment. We had only one room in there.

As Trudy related her father's return, piano music floated in from a neighboring room as if cued, adding to the poignancy of her story.

My father came home after nine months of being in the camp. He came home just half the man he was before, skinny . . . My father had to report to the Gestapo every week about his immigration, and he was in danger. If he wouldn't go away, they would take him back.

They desperately sought a place to which they could escape. Her father had been released from the concentration camp with the understanding he would leave the country. Initially Bolivia looked like a possibility. When Bolivia fell through, they needed to find another path of escape.

So, we waited a little bit, and then they came up with a trip to Shanghai. Shanghai opened and let the Jews come in. But . . . my passport was not ready. My parents had to leave. My parents left in 1939, beginning September, and they said two weeks later goes a second transport to China, Shanghai, and I could be on that boat. But in those two weeks, the war broke out. That's how I was stuck in Germany. That was 1939.

Was a terrible thing for me to be all alone. I had just my uncle and aunt, and I had a cousin. He went with my parents to Shanghai. I later went with his parents, my aunt and uncle, to the concentration camp . . . After six weeks, everybody who was over thirty got taken away and got shot. My uncle and aunt, they were among those people.

Trudy was in ten camps in three-and-a-half years.

And from the ghetto they sent us to many different places to work for a few weeks. A few weeks I was sent with a group of young people to a sugar factory. In that sugar factory, they had big kettles where they cooked the beets to make sugar. They boiled them, and sometimes those kettles boiled over, and we had to wipe off the floors from the boiled-over syrup . . .

At that sugar factory, we stood once in line. They said for delousing. We should bring our blankets. We stood in line maybe for a half hour or longer. All of a sudden, they said we could go home. Later we found out we stood in line to get killed. Why they called it off we never found out.

Another time Trudy was in the hospital and was tipped off to danger by a German nurse.

> *I was about three days in the hospital. There was a nurse who was from Berlin, talked German to me. She said, 'You better get out of here because tomorrow comes an inspector and takes everybody who is sick away.' So, I did get out. Those things happened all the time, where I was that close to die or to getting killed, but I survived.*

No formal liberation led to her release. She and other prisoners awoke in a barn to learn their German captors had run away as the Russians closed in.

> *Some of our women walked away out of that barn . . . they saw Russian soldiers going in their trucks. The soldiers told them, 'You are free, you can go, but don't go that way, go this way,' because the war was not over. It was March 3, 1945. They said, 'You have to be careful not to fall back into German hands' . . . Every night we stayed overnight in a different house, in a different village, and all the villages—this was in Germany—all the villages were empty, the houses. The Germans did run away from the Russians. They left and left everything behind, so we had food.*
>
> *Polish soldiers came . . . they did go through the houses and asking if anybody was sick. I said, 'I'm sick,' and they had a cart, a wagon with cows in front pulling the wagon and take me to the hospital . . . They took me to hospital, and hospital was already taken over by Russians. I had typhoid . . . We called it typhus. I had the highest fever for three days, 105, but the Russians took really good care of us. Shaved our heads. I was seven weeks in the hospital. I remember when they told us the war was over . . . The Russians, they were drinking and dancing and playing their violins. The Russians play—what do they play?* Balalaika! *We were very happy, but I was seven weeks in that hospital. Then I did get out of the hospital.*
>
> *I had two girlfriends; they said, 'Come with us.' I didn't know where to go. I didn't know what to do. Nobody knew.*

Ultimately Trudy was directed to the DP camps:

> *I had a room with two other girls. We got meals. Breakfast, lunch, dinner. Normal. They treated us very good. A few weeks later I met my husband. He lost his whole family in Lvov. His whole family got killed, all of them. He didn't have anybody left.*

Trudy had lost her sister, her grandparents, and her aunt and uncle, but she was more fortunate than some. Her parents had escaped to Shanghai.

> *I tried to find out about my parents. It took me a while. I had an uncle in New York. I couldn't remember his address . . . I find out his address, and I did write to him, and he did send back a letter that my parents are alive and well.*

The most moving part of our interview was when Trudy spoke of receiving that first letter from her parents. Suddenly this event from more than sixty-five years ago was vividly relived before me as if she were experiencing it anew:

> *I was crying, laughing and crying. I was so happy. My mother wrote that she did bake cake and invited all her friends for coffee and cake to celebrate my homecoming.*

Postcard from New Ulm

Trudy and her husband immigrated to Minneapolis after the war. In 1948, her parents joined them.

> *After nine years, not knowing, not hearing anything from each other, being reunited was wonderful, but, of course, my sister was not there. My parents were very happy to be together with me. We found them a little apartment close to ours where we lived on the North Side.*

Trudy and her husband began a family and a new life. They reached out to other survivors who also found homes in the area.

> *Yes, we had a good life here. At first, we had a club here, New Home Club. All the immigrants who came here met there every so often, and we got to meet each other. They were from all over. . . .*
>
> *My parents were quite happy, but my father was a sick man right away when he came. The doctor told him that it could happen at any moment, that he could die. He had a bad heart. But after that he lived six more years. They went on a trip to New Ulm, and there he passed away in the night.*

Trudy paused and leaned forward as if sharing a secret:

> *After the funeral of my father, I got a postcard in the mail from my father, from New Ulm, and he writes, 'We have such a good time, everyone speaks German here . . . and the food is so good, German food.'*

"Born in Germany, raised in Germany," she exclaimed as she threw her hands up in the air, laughing as she related the incongruity of this love of all things German.

I was struck by the fact that Germany was home to them. This country that had turned on them was still so much a part of their culture as expressed through food and language. Its familiarity gave her father comfort to the end.

When Trudy told me the story of her father's death, I knew I had to build the painting around it. This painting incorporates many of the images from Trudy's stories with the postcard from her father as the central image. You can see the German houses that were abandoned, doors open and curtains flying in the wind, as the words of her father on the card emphasize the importance of their German heritage.

I imagined Trudy chasing after that boat to Shanghai, arms raised, holding out her newly printed passport. The monument in the foreground is Herman the German, a statue in New Ulm, a Minnesota town with largely German roots. He raises a sword into the air. Did you notice the stamp on the postcard with the Statue of Liberty raising her torch? Did I plan that? Not consciously. Some synergies just happen.

Sam Saide

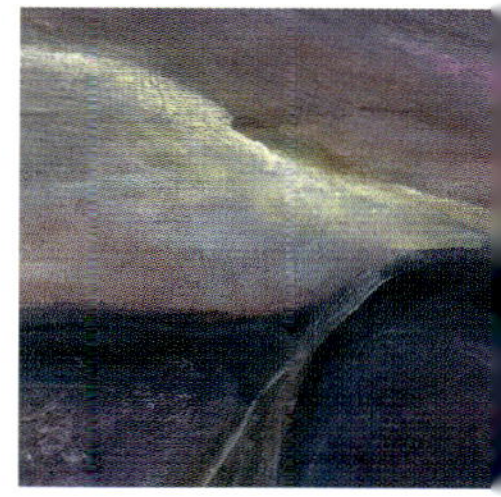

Living by His Wits

We met with Sam Saide in his apartment at Sholom. Sam was short and round, and his round face was topped with a round *kippah*. As he spoke, he paused and repeated himself to ensure we understood him.

Sam was almost thirteen and growing up in Poland when the war broke out. He lost his family and survived by lying about his age. He was sent to build ditches and lay tracks for the railroad.

> *Every three or four weeks they came in, and we had to stand out in a line, and they sort out, and they ask you, 'How old are you?' . . . I was twelve and a half, and I told them I'm eighteen, nineteen, so I was good to work. The rest of them—they had three trucks. They put them on trucks, and when the exhaust pipe come from the bottom up to the top of the roof of the trucks and go inside, that's how they gas them out.*

After several camps, he was sent to Auschwitz-Birkenau, where he was assigned to work in the crematorium. This was not a job one survived. He had an opportunity to get out when the Nazis wanted a transport to go to Warsaw. They didn't want anyone who spoke Polish, but Sam managed to join the transport nonetheless.

> *So I got in between the French and the Italians and the Greeks, and we got into Warsaw . . . The Warsaw ghetto was bombed. People were laying on the basements there like flies.*

Sam explained that he was sent into the destroyed basements where corpses were lying, and he covered them with sand.

> *So, what they did is they blew up the rest of it, the rest of the buildings. Then I had to do clean up* [with] *the bricks . . . The Polish people came in with a horse and a wagon, and they were buying those bricks from the Germans. When they got in, they had to pay so much, and they had to show me a piece of paper: how many bricks they need to buy. So, I gave them the bricks they needed to buy, and sometimes I ask them if they got something, bread or something like that.*
>
> *Pretty soon, they got smart. They brought me a bread, they brought me a salami, and I gave them those bricks. I gave them—instead of twenty bricks—I gave them twenty-five bricks. See, the five bricks, they had a hole on the wagon, and they put it*

in the holder . . . because they count the bricks when they went out. They gave them twenty bricks, and going out they had to show the paper that they got twenty bricks, so they went up on the wagon and count the bricks, twenty bricks, but they didn't count the other ones.

This story stayed with me. It seemed to capture the cold-bloodedness of the Nazis; destroying the ghetto and then selling the remaining bricks to local Poles seemed inconceivable. It also captured the "living by his wits" quality of Sam's experience during the war.

In the background of this painting is the skyline of Warsaw after its destruction. Only a church remained. The sky is dark and hazy. I included the horse and wagon of local Poles purchasing the bricks of a destroyed Jewish culture, as well as Sam loading bricks into the cart. That much-coveted loaf of bread perched on the brick wall is juxtaposed with a similar-sized pile of bricks in Sam's arms, recalling that life-sustaining trade.

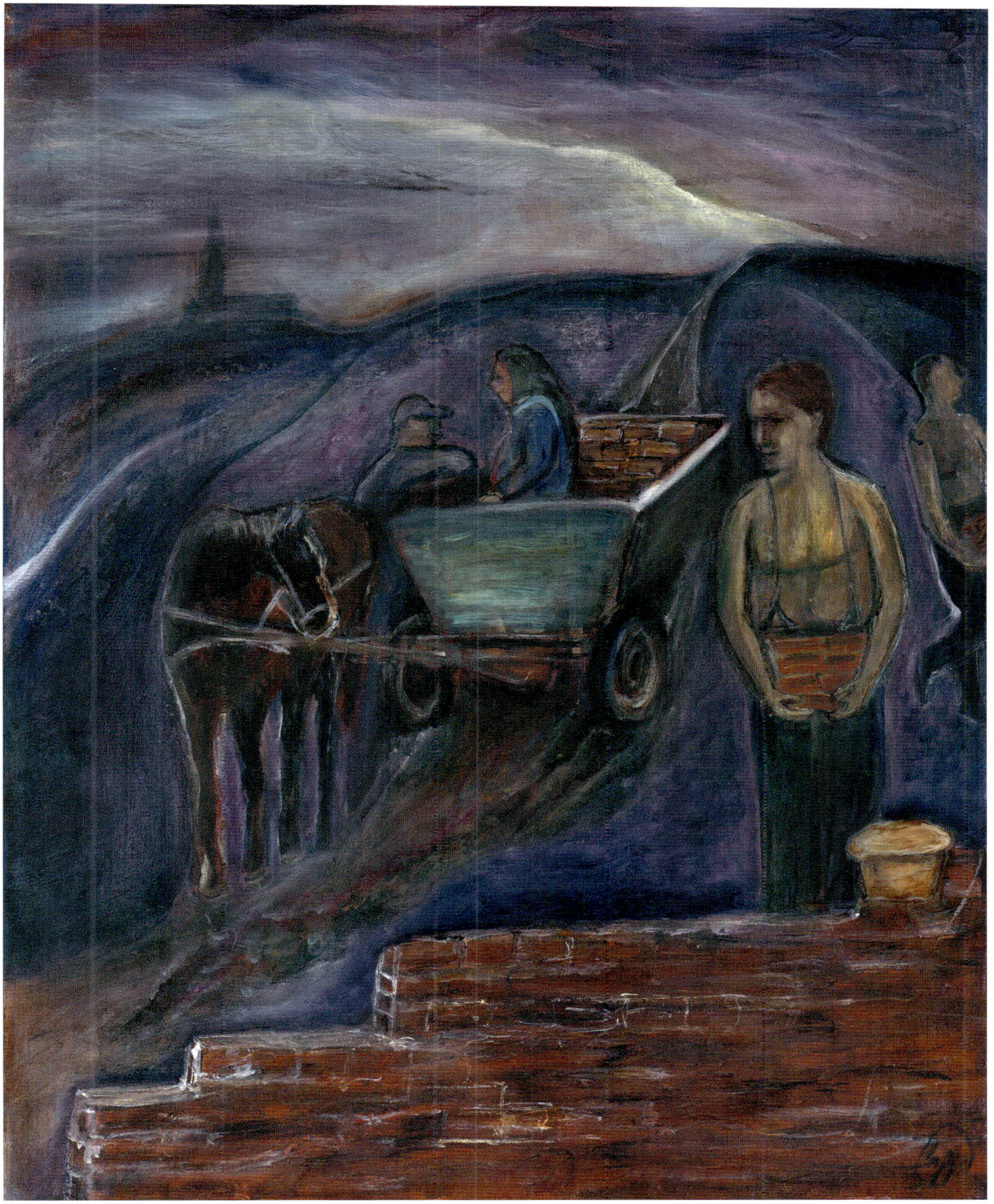

Bricks for Bread, from the story of Sam Saide

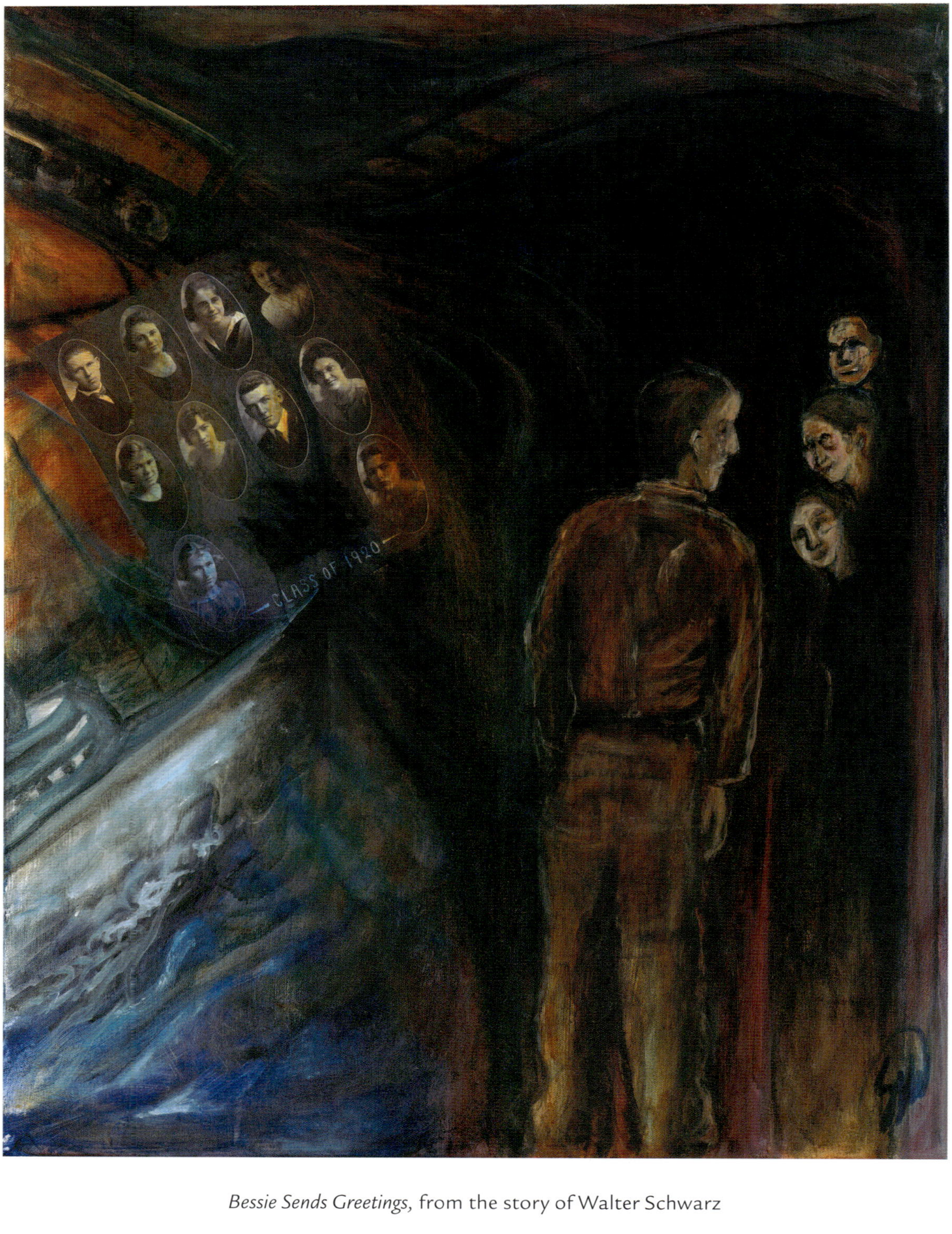

Bessie Sends Greetings, from the story of Walter Schwarz

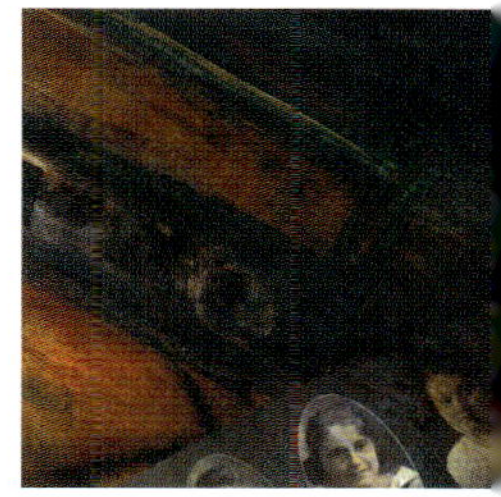

Walter Schwarz

A Narrow Escape

Walter Schwarz was tall with white hair and a distinguished look. His manner was gentle, and he spoke slowly with a cultured accent, laying out his story methodically.

He was fortunate in being able to escape Eastern Europe in the early years of the war. Raised in Romania, he was studying textiles in Czechoslovakia when the Nazis invaded and barred him from his school.

> *I was going to school on March 15, 1935, on the day Germany invaded Czechoslovakia. I was there. My parents were in Romania . . . I went to school on that day. The place was full of German army, the post office and the city hall was already occupied by the German army. They had sentries in front . . . I walked up the steps of the school. I saw by the entrance there were a bunch of hoodlums with swastikas.* 'Juden raus' [Jews out]. *They wouldn't let any Jews into that school . . .*
>
> *The Jewish students were meeting in a park not far from the school, so I joined them, and there was a rally. We were wondering: what should we do now? One of the student leaders . . . urged all the Jewish students to get out of town, as fast as you can, as far away as you can . . . I went and packed my bags. The railroads were already run by the German army, so I had to get permission to buy a ticket . . . It happened to be a sympathetic officer . . . so I was able to buy a ticket . . . I believe that was the last train that left Czechoslovakia* [for Romania].

Walter left Eastern Europe with his family because of his mother's experience in the United States. Her father had brought the whole family to the US, and she was brought up and educated in America from age five. She returned to Europe as a young woman, to marry.

> *At that time in 1939, the war started already, and Czechoslovakia was already occupied, and Romania was going to be next . . . My parents made frantic efforts to get out. And the Romanian quota—they were on a quota system: so many, but not more.*
>
> *Because of her* [his mother's] *background in America—she went to school here; she was not a citizen because she was a child, but her parents were citizens—she had to show evidence to the American Consulate that she had been in America. By chance, her sister who lived in America was a good friend of her former teacher, and she once*

met her and asked her, 'Is there any evidence that my sister Bessie was your student?' She says she has a class picture. So, she presented that class picture and said, 'This is Bessie here.' So, my mother had to show that picture to the American Consulate and said, 'This is me, I was there.' . . . And she spoke perfect English, of course. She had gone to school here. And on that basis, she was able to get a visa to get all her whole family in . . .

When my family got out, we boarded a ship in Genoa, Italy . . . That was the last refugee ship that left Italy. On the way to the United States, Italy declared war on France in 1940. Germany was already in the thick of it, but Italy wanted to get in on it, and so they thought the easiest way was to attack France. So they declared war on France. And from then on, they dropped the refugees off in New York, and the ship went back empty back to Italy . . .

A Ritchie Boy

I was anxious to get back at the Germans. I visited the army recruiting station and said, 'Will you take me?'

I was not a citizen, and they said, 'No, if you are not a citizen, we can't take you.'

A year later was Pearl Harbor, and then they would take foreigners. In 1942, I was drafted into the army. So, after I was drafted, it took only about a month of service, military training service. After about a month, they made me a citizen. . . .

At that time, the army was combing their military camps for people who spoke German, and they found me, and one day the captain of my company called me into his office and said, 'Go pack up your duffle bag, you're shipping out.' . . .

I put my duffle bag in the truck, and we went overnight to Camp Ritchie, Maryland. Camp Ritchie was a basic training camp for people who spoke German. About 90% of the people were people of the same background as mine, refugees from Central Europe, and they all spoke German. They had to speak English, too, of course. And so, that's where I got my training.

There he was taught to interrogate prisoners of war. Those who served as interrogators from Camp Ritchie became known as "Ritchie Boys" and shared a sense of brotherhood.

Walter is a very gentle person. It was hard for his children to imagine him interrogating German prisoners. His daughter Sylvia laughed, "We used to joke that if he had a prisoner who wasn't giving information, he would use the harshest technique he knew, which was to go 'Tsk' and walk away. That would cow anybody into giving information."

After the war, Walter was stationed in Czechoslovakia where his story had begun.

> *Every time we went by jeep through a town, I saw in the middle of the town there was a big bulletin board, and people were gathering around there. I said, 'What are they looking for?' You know, gathering around the bulletin board. This was a time when the concentration camps were being liberated, and the International Red Cross published the names of the people who were released, and they put them on the bulletin board. Of course, everybody wanted to see who's coming home and who's not coming home . . .*
>
> *My mother had a lot of relatives who were sent to the concentration camps, and she got hold of one of those lists, and she found a name that she knew that was a second cousin of hers . . . He had just been released from Theresienstadt, and he was coming home . . . My mother wrote to me, 'Would it be possible for* [you] *to visit that family?'*

Walter recounted his visit to his newly-found relatives.

> *I found the address, and I knocked on the door, rang the bell. The people came to the door, slightly opening it. What is a man in uniform doing here? They were suspicious of people in uniform anyway. So, they opened the door, and I addressed them in German and I said, 'Bessie Schwarz, my mother, is sending you greetings.'*
>
> *As soon as I said that, then of course they hugged and kissed me, and I was welcomed into the house. And then they told me the story. Now this was a father, a mother and a fifteen-year-old daughter. Only the father went to the concentration camp. Why? He was Jewish, and they were not. But at that time it didn't matter, they took the non-Jews also and put them in concentration camps. In this case, he got a divorce before he left to save his wife and daughter . . .*

I was intrigued with the idea of the cracked door with family members peering out and moving from suspicion to joy. Walter's experience as a Ritchie Boy was an important part of his legacy, so I wanted to do an image with him in uniform. There was a directionality in his story, forced out of Czechoslovakia at the beginning of the war and then returning there as a Ritchie Boy. I was also struck by the chanciness of his escape: the last boat, the last train, and a school picture all figured in the story. While the school picture that is collaged into the painting isn't the actual image, it is from the same time period. You can find these elements in the painting.

A Few Thoughts

Each of the survivors I interviewed lost family to the Holocaust. In each case, their own survival, while in part due to actions they took, also involved elements of chance. Had Hanna's mother not sent her to London, she would have shared her family's fate in Auschwitz. Had Trudy not been alerted to leave the hospital by a German nurse, her death would have been assured. If Sam, as a young boy, hadn't had the wit to lie about his age, he would have faced certain death, and had Walter's mother not been able to prove her past in the United States, his family would not have been able to get out.

Each shared the resourcefulness to build a new life in a new country. They entered the United States as young adults, eager to embark on the experiences of young adulthood that had been displaced by the war. They began new careers, often while still mastering the language. Sam's skill at living by his wits during the war soon transferred to making a living. Hanna found important supports in her aunt and uncle as she finished her nursing education and found work as a nurse. Trudy, with her husband who was also a survivor, happily reunited with her parents and built ties with other survivors. Walter, as a veteran whose family had successfully come to the United States on the cusp of the war, established his career, married, and began to raise a family. Marrying and raising a family was an important theme for each of these survivors, emblematic of their new beginning.

Jews from the USSR

Jews from the USSR had lived with active antisemitism. Religious practice was suppressed, especially that of Judaism. For some, food, song, and story became central in carrying their heritage forward. Elders from the Soviet Union generally left to follow their children. Their children had left to escape antisemitism and create a better life for *their* children. Some immigrated in the 1970s. Many more came in the 1990s, after the fall of the former Soviet Union.

Many of these stories include both the Holocaust and military service. The Soviet Union suffered what is believed to be 26.6 million deaths during WWII, and that loss looms large for all who lived through it.[8] The Holocaust was particularly significant for Jews in the western republics that were occupied by the Nazis, more than for Jews in the Russian Soviet Socialist Republic. My interviewees, who came from the Ukraine and Belarus, lost much family. Many survived through military service or by relocating to more secure parts of the USSR.

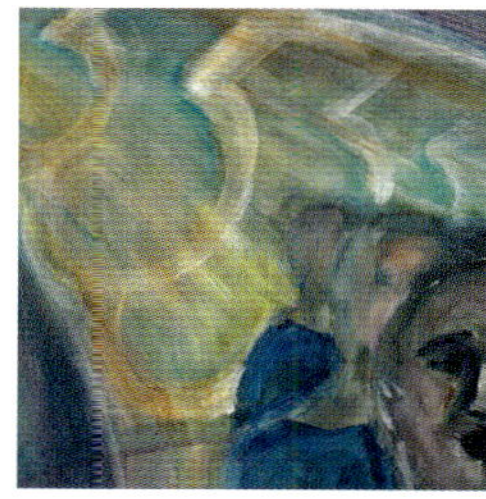

Rakhil Sheynkman

A History Lesson

Rakhil Sheynkman had a round face and laughing eyes. She had a big personality and conveyed it quite emphatically through facial expressions and body language. When the English language presented a barrier, Rakhil used her hands to extend the reach of her vocabulary.

Rakhil began by talking about her parents, who lived in Kiev, providing a bit of a history lesson:

> *They moved to Kiev in 1911 after they got married . . . and there was a famous district in Kiev that was called Podol. The district Podol was where all of the Jewish craftsmen lived. They were not allowed to live in the center of the city, so that area was designated for those who were not allowed. Wealthy Jews . . . were allowed to sell and trade in Kreshchatyk . . . a more central area of Kiev. The craftsmen from Podol supplied them with goods . . .*
>
> *When I was growing up, Ukrainians and Jews got along great. We never felt any antisemitism . . . We always exchanged all the goodies, all the treats for holidays . . . Our home was always open to all the Russian Ukrainian neighbors, and the same thing, we were always welcome in their homes.*
>
> [That began to change in] *1933 when the hunger was coming, the* Holodomor. *It was the hunger, the starvation when all of the harvests were killed, and it was . . . artificially-brought starvation basically, when thousands and thousands . . . of people were killed . . . by killing the harvests and crops . . .*
>
> *Antagonism was . . . created because Jews knew how to survive. Being craftsmen and tradesmen, they knew how to survive in these hardest times. Ukrainians and Russians did not fare so well. So, it created jealousy and antagonism and . . . this led to antisemitism.*
>
> [The Jews] *had a natural wit and skill to fare better because they knew how to use every piece. A piece of chicken that the Jewish woman would buy—she would cut it up to the very last inch and would sell the inside parts and the wings separately and the legs separately, and she would make more money by selling that chicken and getting more for the family that they could live on as opposed to just bringing it home and cooking it up.*
>
> *The Jewish boys would come to the beach, and they would sell plain cold water for*

a kopek, a penny, and people were buying it for just a kopek . . . They were more entrepreneurial . . . They knew how to survive, and they had that natural wit.

The Jewish people . . . they opened their own shops, the leather man, the watch man, the hat people, the dressmakers, they all started opening up their shops and started living quite well, and that could not but bring a lot of jealousy and hostility.

The rich Ukrainians would open up shops in the center of the city, and they would hire all these Jewish craftspeople to come work for them, like furriers, and watch men and hat men.

It's just that all this jealousy and hostility began when the hunger struck because Ukrainians could not survive, and they had to blame someone.

A War Hero

Our second interview was in Rakhil's apartment and included Rakhil's daughter, Liana Ravkin. Family photos sat atop furniture, and Rakhil drew our attention to one of her wearing many medals from her service in WWII. This was an important part of her identity.

> *I weighed my options and decided that since I had relatives in Kharkov, I'd go there . . . and volunteer for active duty. I was then assigned to be a communications expert. I worked in communications and made it all the way to Berlin.*
>
> *I was part of the Stalingrad battle, and I was wounded. I have a scar* [she touched the center of her forehead] . . . *from that battle . . . I lost my eyesight in my right eye.*
>
> *The relatives . . . from my mother's home town, 28 people . . . they came looking for shelter . . . They were told that nothing was going to happen to Kiev, that the Russians would hold the Germans at bay and nothing would happen to Kiev . . . The Ukrainian neighbors told us that they were sent to Babi Yar* [a site in Kiev where almost 50,000 Jews were massacred].

Liana spoke of how the experience of WWII touched the Russians, far more than the Americans.

> *See it was such a huge thing for Soviet Union, period. Because we were involved, Soviet Union, in war. So much. It touched actually almost every family. It was completely different than in United States. It was on our territory, number one. You had Pearl*

Harbor, a little piece, and the rest was in Europe and Japan or somewhere on the Asia part. For us it was on our land, and everybody was at war

Liana was proud of her mother's heroism and knew her stories.

When . . . Soviet army, started liberating Poland, she went with the army to Majdanek, to Oswiecim. She saw all these mounds of people's glasses, of people's purses, of people's teeth. Mattresses with people's hair, that's what she saw with her own eyes. She came when chambers were still working.

Becoming a Citizen

Rakhil Sheynkman and her daughter, Liana, immigrated from Kiev. Liana came first with her husband and son in the late 1980s, and then Rakhil followed several years later. They left the Soviet Union to seek a life free of antisemitism.

When Rakhil came to America, she wanted to become a citizen right away. Liana chuckled as she recalled the conversation.

She was seventy-five when she came here, and she said, 'I have to be citizen'

I said, 'Ok, Mother, let's learn English a little bit.' So, she learned . . .

As Liana told this story, she turned to ask her mother a question in Russian. Rakhil thought for a long moment, took a deep breath, and declared, "Memorial Day ees holiday."

Liana then explained how Rakhil went for her citizenship interview with an immigration official to show she could speak English.

She learned how to write it. He was amazed because she came and she said, 'I am Rakhil Sheynkman' and she said how old is she—she understood, we learned, we were learning all of it—and where she lived. 'Good for you. Good for you,' he said to her. And she said her address in English. Then she wrote, 'Memorial Day is a holiday.' It was the best thing he'd ever seen probably.

Rakhil held her fingers in big circles around her eyes, imitating how the immigration official had looked at her, in amazement.

Food, Song, and Story

Rakhil had fond recollections of her childhood. She grew up in Kiev in a family with six children. While her parents were not observant, they kept kosher and fasted on Yom Kippur. The children attended a Jewish school and spoke Yiddish at home. She remembered their special Shabbat dinner of sweet and sour beef, *kugel, kikhl* (cookies) and *challah.*

Food and song were central themes, and her mother was a significant figure in her memories, the cement of the family. Rakhil still makes her mother's recipes. When religion could no longer be practiced, food and song became the means of transferring tradition.

When asked about legacy she responded:

> *Optimism, dancing, singing, stories . . . That's the legacy . . . and cooking . . . Around the table, she* [her mother] *always started singing, and all the children and family sang along with her.*

Liana told the story of a recipe that has made its way through many generations.

> *You know, gefilte fish, my mom carried from my grandma, and I never even started it yet, but she promised me she would teach me—she would give me the recipe—but gefilte fish was the best. She does it from recipe of her mother, and her mom had it from her mom, so it is a very secret recipe.*

Liana interpreted for Rakhil, as Rakhil's hands went through the motions of shaping the gefilte fish.

> *She says that here what she sees, it's not the right gefilte fish. It's like a meatball, long. It's not the right thing. You have to have fish and stuff it with the meat,* 'gefilte'*—stuffed . . .*
>
> *So you cut the fish, you take the meat out, you grind it with the spices and everything, and then when this grinded fish meat is ready, you put it in the fish skin. Fill it. And then you put it on the many hours to steam . . . It's a long procedure. People don't have time anymore. It's better to go to Costco to buy it.*

Recipes were not the only things shared. Rakhil was born right after the revolution, a time Liana described as:

> *An era of atheism—any religions, including Jewish religion, were persecuted, and Jewish religion especially . . . So my mom . . . knew about Jewish holidays from her mom. Myself, whatever my mom remembered she told me, but we couldn't go* [to the synagogue].

In Liana's lifetime, it was dangerous to go to the synagogue if they valued their futures.

> *We had one synagogue . . . One, which was attended probably by older people who have nothing to lose, retired people, people who didn't work. For younger people— I could lose my university. I could lose my job. I could lose everything if I would be* [identified], *and I would be because it was all kind of monitored, who's going there, who's coming.*

Secondhand Kind of Person

Liana attempted to explain the antisemitism that ultimately drove them out of the Soviet Union:

> *It's hard to understand for people who never live there. You just kind of learn with years, you learn to live with it. You just know that you are secondhand kind of person, and certain fields, certain places, you will never be able to get to.*

"You can't get the good job being Jewish," says Rakhil.

Liana explains:

> *For example, . . . my son was . . . teased to be Jew. Then we put him to school where . . .* [there were] *more Jewish kids than the school . . .next to us. And actually, I want him to go to the school with English language, specialized . . . I came* [to] *the director of the school, the superintendent, and she said after children are supposed to finish this school, they are having certificate of interpreters, and usually it is military interpreters.*
>
> *And she said, 'We can get your son into the school, but he will never get the certificate.'*
>
> *I said, 'Why?'*
>
> *And she said, 'Because you are Jewish. Don't you understand?'*
>
> *When I graduated from university, it was hard for me to find a job. And you have to call somebody, to know somebody . . . Because for Jewish people it wasn't possible.*

Liana explained that the passport was a person's ID, and it revealed one's nationality.

> *When you go to work, when you, for example, go to interview for a job, they look at your passport. It say*[s] *'Jewish.' We're not Russians or Soviets. Everybody has a known nationality, so if you're Lithuanian, but live in Ukraine it says 'Lithuanian.' If*

you are Russian it says 'Russian,' if you are Ukrainian it says 'Ukrainian.' If you are Jew it says 'Jew.' It's a line number 5, and everybody says, 'Is your line number 5 ok?' It means 'Are you Jewish or not?' If you are Jewish it will be a big question.

Liana expressed her surprise at being called Russian in the United States.

You see we've been all of our lives Jews. In America, we become Russians. . . . We're Russian, but we're not. We're from Russia, but we've never been Russian. We've always been Jews. Jews here and Jews there. But here we're Americans, American Jew. Over there we were just Jew. Period.

When I thought of Rakhil's story, I was struck by how much of her tradition was an oral one shared through family traditions. Rakhil had spoken of how her mother would lead them in song at the table during Pesach, singing Yiddish songs she had learned from her mother. Rakhil in turn sang some of these for us. Similarly, Rakhil had learned how to make gefilte fish from her mother, who had learned from Rakhil's grandmother. The thread that echoed throughout was the handing down of knowledge and tradition, shared through food and song and story, even when the practice of religion wasn't possible.

When I painted this, I imagined a long arc of women trailing into the distance, figuratively sharing the same table in song, collapsing time through their shared traditions. I gave each of them a Star of David necklace to wear proudly, something they could not have done in the Soviet Union. The Kiev synagogue stands in the background.

The number 5 is included to remind us of Line 5 on the former Soviet passport, identifying one as Jewish and thus marked for discrimination. Here it becomes a metaphor for the many generations of Jews who lived under antisemitism throughout Russian history.

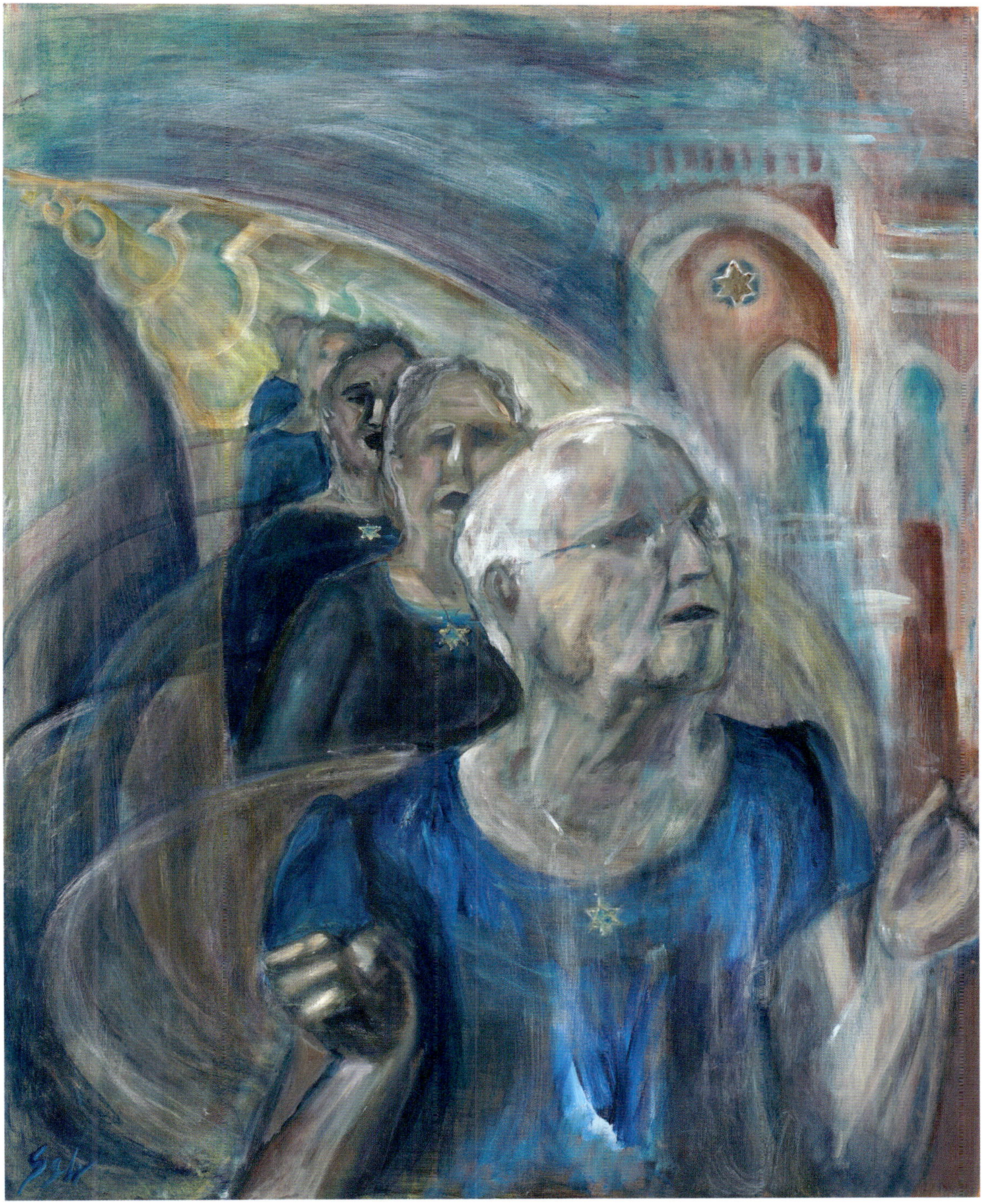

From Her Mother, from the story of Rakhil Sheynkman

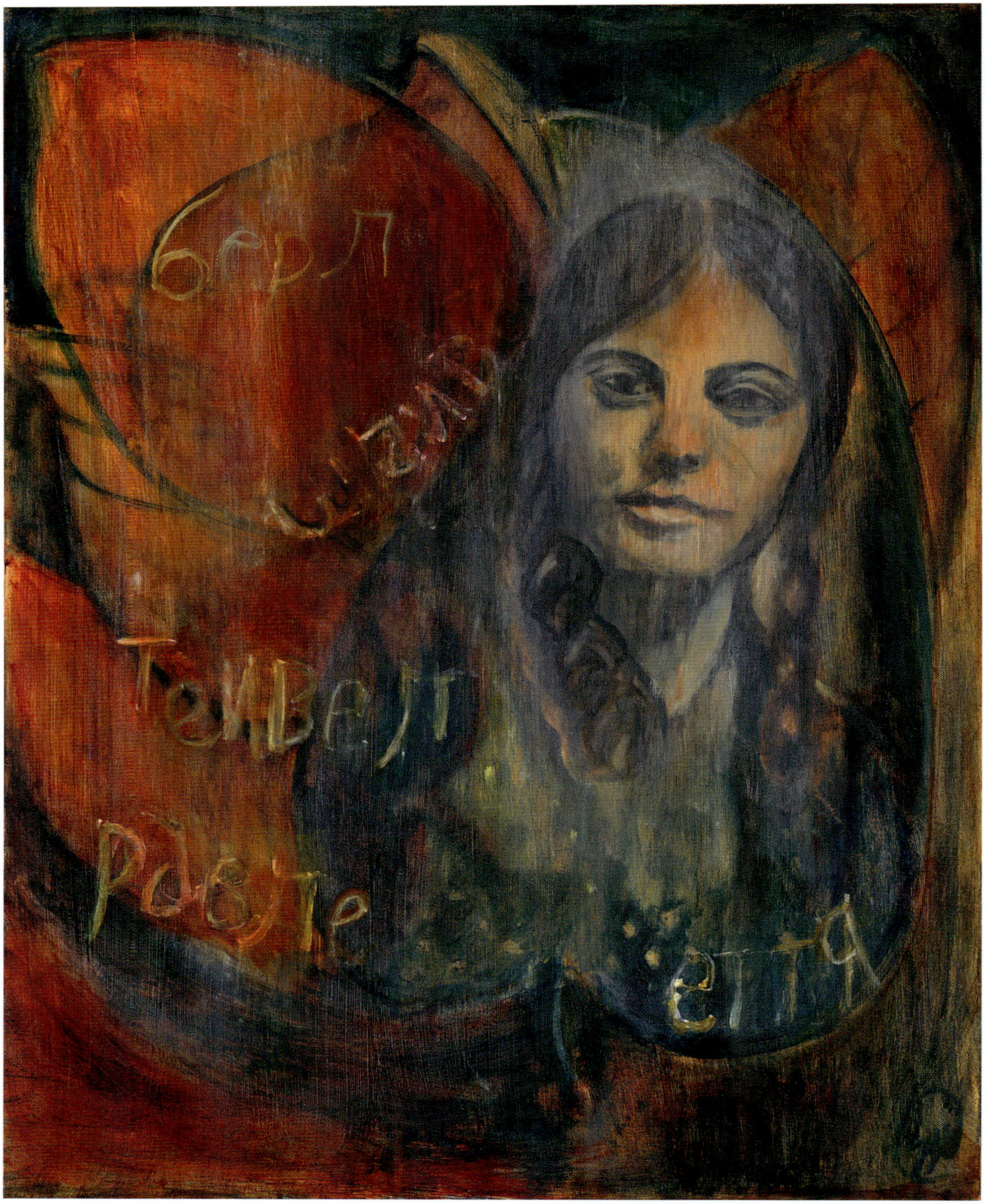

Fallen Leaves, from the story of Boris Lerner

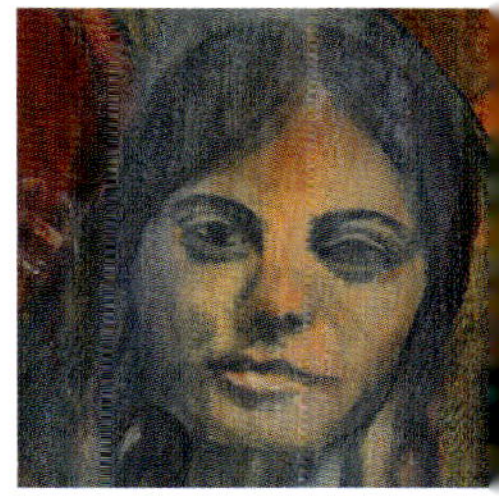

Boris Lerner

A Child Survivor

When I began an interview, I would start with a family history, names of parents, siblings, spouses, children, when they were born, when they died. When I asked Boris Lerner when his mother died, he replied, "She was shot when she was thirty-nine." Boris was seven years old at the time. I knew this would not be an easy interview.

Of the elders, Boris Lerner was our youngest interviewee. That is, of course, a relative term as most were in their nineties, while Boris was on the threshold of eighty. In front of him were family photos he had brought to share. He had a somber air about him, that of a serious person. I was to learn that he had lived a sobering life. Boris was a child during the Holocaust and saw much of his family murdered. Later he followed his only child to the United States.

Before the war, Boris lived in Mogilev Podolsk in the Ukraine with his parents and four siblings. He was named after his grandfather who was a cantor in the synagogue. Both his grandparents and his parents were religious. They attended synagogue and celebrated Jewish holidays. Before Shabbat and holidays, his grandmother came to help his mother prepare. Boris remembered that Shabbat dinner was often boiled chicken with beans and broth, baked strudel and *leckach,* a honey cake. His parents spoke Yiddish, but his mother spoke Ukrainian and Russian to the children. Only his grandmother spoke Yiddish to the grandchildren. While his oldest brother finished *cheder,* the other children went to the Ukrainian school. As he recalled his family together, Boris spoke lovingly of his beautiful mother in her red beret.

And then his childhood ended.

> *When the war broke out, we were put into a ghetto . . . We had to survive somehow in the ghetto, and the Nazis, the Germans, warned us that if we make one step outside of the ghetto we will be instantly executed. My father had many friends among the Ukrainians. They helped, and they brought food to help us survive. From the ghetto we were taken to the concentration camp . . .*
>
> [My family was among those] *building a bunker for Hitler. When they finished the project, they were all executed.*
>
> *My father and my two sisters were working on the same project. I was there also,*

but not involved in the construction as I was too young . . . I witnessed the murder of my family and helped to pick up the bodies.

We were scheduled to be shot because we were useless, my aunt who was pregnant and the older people . . . We were loaded onto open trucks, and as we were leaving to be shot, a German officer . . . stopped the truck and said the site was not ready for the execution . . . My aunt realized that we had to run. Someone pointed her to a man who helped to lead people out of the camp . . . She had gold coins sewn [into her clothing], *and she made arrangements, paying with those coins* [to] *the man who would take us out . . .*

I was unconscious because I was beaten severely and I lost consciousness . . . so the woman—because my aunt couldn't carry me—the woman who helped to carry me, she had paid for that woman, for me and for herself to be taken out of the concentration camp. We were taken outside of the camp . . . We started walking, in the middle of the night, and some peasants . . . hid us for a day or two days . . . That's how we made it to Mogilev Podolsk . . . We were caught and sent back to the camp, but by that time the Germans did away with everyone in the concentration camp and the Red army marched in, and we were freed . . .

The camp was liberated in 1944, the year Boris turned 12. With no family, he was sent to an orphanage.

[After the war] *I was in the orphanage and went to school . . . There were some recruiters who came to the orphanage, and they said they were representatives of America. They offered to put us on a ship and be taken to America. I got a letter in the orphanage in Mogilev Podolsk . . . that my brother was alive . . . That's why I did not go with the rest of the children who chose to travel to America. I was hoping to meet up with my brother. Many children left, and they perished because the ship sank.*

Ultimately Boris reconnected with his brother and his sister. Both had survived because they had been drafted. He received a letter from each of them, telling him they would take care of him. He later attended school in Moscow where he became an engineering specialist and married.

Boris came to the United States in 1993, following his son. He noted that his son was mocked and harassed in the USSR because he was Jewish. That environment affected their choice of surname.

My last name was Lerner, and my son was also Lerner, but then my mother-in-law and my wife, they began to doubt that it is not right that we have written our child with a Jewish last name . . . We decide together to give him the [not Jewish] *last name of my wife . . .*

When he came to America, he changed the last name back. He became Lerner.

Antisemitism was not a new development in Russia, nor were efforts to avoid it. Boris related the story of his father-in-law whose father had become a Christian before the revolution:

> *They did it because they couldn't work, and they couldn't study. They couldn't do nothing. They need to change the nationality. In Russia, to live in Leningrad, to live in Moscow—it was in the nineteenth century—Jewish people have to change their nationality . . .*
>
> *When the revolution came in Russia, my father-in-law, he came to the police, and he told them that now he doesn't need to be a Christian . . . instantly he is Jewish. And in the passport of his parents, was written that they are Christian.*
>
> *They used to go to the church, and after the church they used to come to home, and they used to pray Jewish. It was a system. If you would like to be a scientist, if you would like to be a lawyer, if you would like to be an engineer, if you would like to live in Leningrad, if you would like to live in Moscow, you have to be not Jewish. You have to be Christian . . .*
>
> *My wife was considered Russian, but the face was Jewish. She was often questioned because she looked so Jewish nobody believed she was indeed Russian . . . When we got married, we decided to make our son's life easier, and he was registered as Russian, but he also looked Jewish, and he was teased anyway.*

When I asked Boris about legacy, he replied,

> *I want young people to remember what had happened to me and my family in the past, but I also want to warn that all the Jewish trouble is not over. I don't know what's going to happen to Israel. I want Jewish youth to be proud of who they are and carry the legacy of the people who had died because they were Jewish. I'm concerned about very strong assimilation . . . I'm doing this in memory of my family who were shot and killed, tortured by the Nazis.*

After the war, Boris sought a picture of family members and was only able to find a school picture of his sister, Ettya, a sepia-colored picture set in a leaf shape. That became my inspiration for painting Boris's story.

I decided to echo that form in additional leaves with the names of his family members who perished. I wanted the image to be muted, as if seen through the glass of memory.

Yevgeniy Mazo

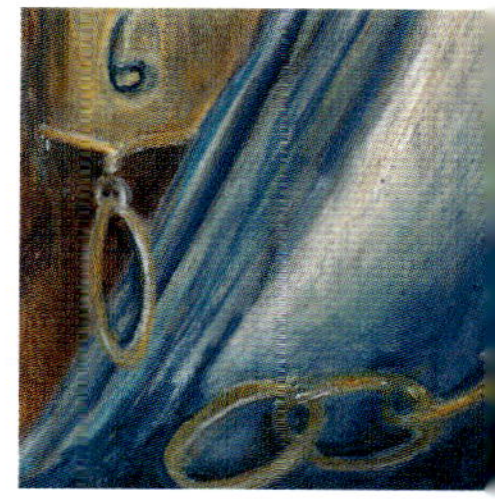

Unchained Legacy

Yevgeniy Mazo came to our interview with several books in hand, all ones he had written exploring branches of his family. He chuckled as he related his stories; a sly smile stole across his face as he waited for his ironic humor to be revealed in translation. His eyes echoed his bemusement.

[I am from] *a small town, a* shtetl, *called Bykhov in Mogilev region in Belarus.*

My grandfather married when he was 14 and my grandmother was 12. They were still playing in the sandbox, and kerosene was very expensive so they had 18 children. They went to bed early.

My mother was the youngest, and she was the most beautiful, she claimed. My father was born in Minsk and was stationed in the army in Bykhov. He saw my mother, fell in love, and moved her to Minsk . . . we moved to Minsk when I was one year old, so I lived all my life in Minsk . . .

In 1934, my father decided to look for happiness in Birobidzhan . . . He left the family, gave me three rubles, and said that should be enough for my life, and I never saw him again . . .

I went on my summer vacations . . . to the family when I was little. My grandfather and all the others were peddlers there. There were like 18 carriages; all the cousins came to pick me up at the railway station. Everybody wanted to take me, but I loved to stay with my grandfather.

He was a very wise man. He had lacquered patent leather boots. The day he was scheduled to die, he decided. He had a vest with a golden chain, with a watch. He told me, 'I'm going to die, and you're going to inherit this watch,' and I couldn't wait . . . to get that watch. I loved to stay with him. My grandfather, before he died, he called me and said [to] *go get the daughter, and the daughter gathered the whole* [family] *in his house. And he said, 'Children, I'm dying.' They were all surprised and said, 'You're going to live for another 100 years.' He was 99 years and 8 months. 'No, children.' He kind of gave us a riddle that it's time to go. He drank a little wine and turned to the wall and died . . .*

Among all the siblings, from 18 children they had 294 children in Bykhov. When Germans came to Bykhov, there was a castle that belonged to a Polish count. They gathered all the Jews and all my cousins, and they were all shot there in that castle.

When I was on a business trip in Berlin I met this old German man and asked him where he was during the war, and he said he was in a concentration camp. And I thought it could have been him who had shot 200 relatives . . .

Because I was in Minsk, I survived and was drafted and went to serve . . . I was heavily wounded . . . I served on the Leningrad front. The Germans claimed that they didn't want to waste ammunition . . . because the inhabitants of Leningrad were going to starve to death anyway. Seven hundred thousand people perished from hunger in Leningrad. So . . . my unit defended the Leningrad line.

After the war, Yevgeniy became a journalist and worked for a publishing house as an editor. He encountered antisemitism there but seemed quite matter of fact about it, as if it were nothing out of the ordinary. That was the world to which he was accustomed.

I was a senior editor, and on Lenin's birthday they would ordinarily give raises. I would not get one. I knew why. I was an honor guard when one of the prominent journalists . . . passed away, and I was told not to be on the honor guard because I was Jewish, and they wanted only Russians there. It was nothing significant.

Yevgeniy's eldest son, a doctor, had immigrated to America first. This son then insisted on his father coming to America right away to address health problems. Yevgeniy had surgery shortly after arriving.

Yevgeniy authored many books, and the stories he told me had a somewhat magical quality to them. Many were stories he had gathered and recorded about his family. He told me of his relationship to the Spanish artist Juan Bautista Martinez del Mazo, who married Diego Velasquez's daughter, and about the chief rabbi of Moscow, Rabbi Jacob Maze. This rabbi was a Mazo family member who had testified for the Beilis defense when a Jew was falsely accused of ritual murder of Christian children. Yevgeniy concluded with the story of the original Mazo, who arrived in Russia with Napoleon's army. Ultimately, that Mazo had married a Belarussian woman and settled in Mazozhen, the town of Yevgeniy's father.

There were so many unusual stories that I wasn't quite sure how to represent Yevgeniy. I went back to the beginning, to the story about visiting his grandfather as a child. As this project was about legacy, I decided to paint the lost legacy. You will see the carriages of Yevgeniy's family members greeting him at the train station and his grandfather's watch with just a portion of its gold chain. Note the broken link, representing lost family. On either side, you will find the pages of a book, carrying us away in story. In the sky, you can find the suggestion of three rubles, the legacy from his father.

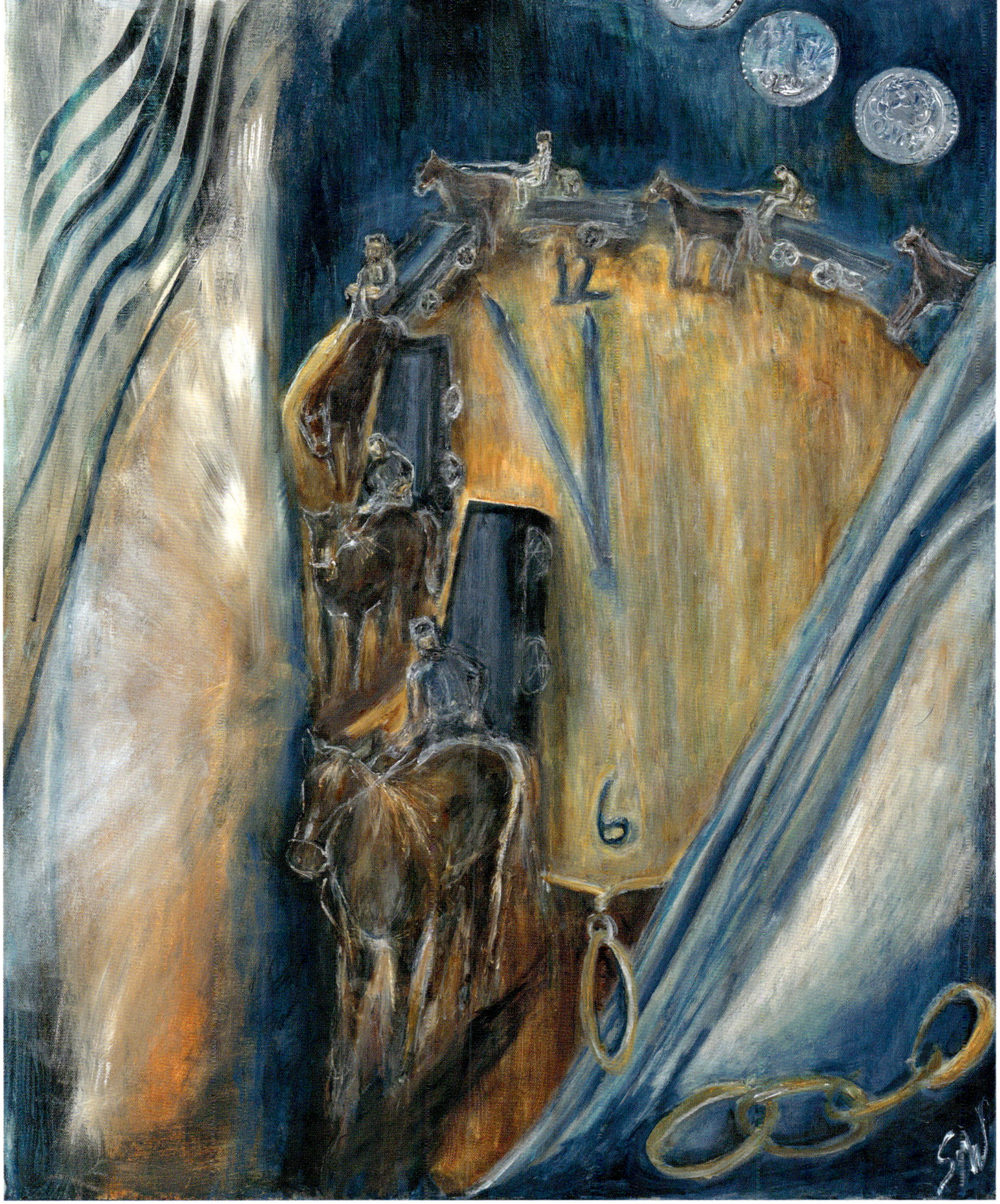

Unchained Legacy, from the story of Yevgeniy Mazo

A Few Thoughts

Several immigrants from the former Soviet Union spoke at length of the antisemitism they experienced there. They often expressed concerns about the treatment of their children in the Soviet Union. They were older at the time of their immigration; as a result, their experience was different from that of the survivors who had immigrated before them. In most cases their children decided to leave first, to find better opportunities for *their* children. As parents and grandparents, these elders followed soon after.

They lacked exposure to most practices of Judaism, but many took pleasure in watching their children rediscover those long-forgotten roots. In my interview with Rakhil, she sang many songs to us that she had learned as a child, when her mother led the family in song. When a musician visited Sholom, I watched Rakhil and others join in with enthusiasm. They knew all the Yiddish words and took comfort in the familiarity of the music that connected them to their history. Both Yevgeniy and Rakhil had served in the military. While Boris was too young to participate in that way, he was drafted into a far more personal war, witnessing the destruction of his much-loved family.

After the war, each was called upon to rebuild his or her life. They carved out careers, raised families, and—when the opportunity presented itself—sought refugee status, following the path of their children. Despite the frequent barrier of language, each conveyed a distinctive personality. Yevgeniy was a storyteller with a wry wit; Boris spoke of honoring his family's memory, even as he voiced concerns about the future; Rakhil expressed herself emphatically through song and gesture.

The Living Archive

As a genealogist, I have a love of history, not just as dry documents, but as an opportunity to uncover story. While learning about my interviewees, I often did genealogy research on their lives, tracing their journey to the United States, matching their life story to the documents that accompanied it. I also spent time in the Nathan and Theresa Berman Upper Midwest Jewish Archives, exploring the Jewish history of this region and how it touched their experiences. As I immersed myself in the history, I realized that Sholom was no less an archive, albeit a living one. The stories from my interview with Dorothy Brochin Wittcoff, about her father's store, married up with archive documents about her father and recollections of her late brother, Ben Brochin. Even Brochin's, the store, was documented in archives detailing its purchases of matzo and herring. In the archives, I discovered a young Fannie Schanfield, when she was president of Hadassah in the 1960s,[9] now one of my interviewees fifty years later, in her nineties. History is ultimately preserved in such archives, but through this project I had an opportunity to bring it to life.

Certain themes emerged through the interviews, themes that often define the Jewish experience: antisemitism, community, and immigration.

Antisemitism

Many of our interviewees had fled antisemitism in Europe. Whether it was pogroms, the Holocaust, or the discrimination of the USSR, all were seeking a better life free of antisemitism. In many cases that was not what they found, for until the middle of the twentieth century, a very visible antisemitism was often widely accepted in the US. There was a reason so much of the Jewish population in Minneapolis was self-employed and provided services and products within the Jewish community. It was difficult to get a job outside the community if you were Jewish.

Initially many Jews just accepted this as the normal course. It was consistent with their experience in Europe, so they had come to expect it. Even by the late 1930s, help-wanted ads read "Gentile Preferred." Some Jews passed as non-Jews, some changed their names, and still others found ways to be enterprising within the Jewish community.[10]

Many of the large corporations within the city would not interview Jewish applicants. After Hubert H. Humphrey became mayor in 1945, he did a study that found "63% of all Minneapolis firms hired no blacks, Jews or Japanese Americans." In 1947, a city ordinance outlawed the denial of employment based on race, creed, or color, but a further study by the Federation of Women Teachers of Minneapolis found that job discrimination continued nonetheless.[11]

In 1946, an article by Carey McWilliams addressed the deep-rooted antisemitism of Minneapolis, describing an "iron curtain" that separated Jews from non-Jews. McWilliams noted that Jews were excluded from the civic life of the city, ineligible for membership in organizations such as the Kiwanis, Rotary, Lions, or Toastmasters. Even the Automobile Club excluded Jews. As noted earlier, McWilliams referred to Minneapolis as "the capitol [*sic*] of antisemitism in the United States."[12]

Minneapolis was markedly different than its sister city across the river. In Minneapolis, the major industries of milling, lumber, transportation, banking, and insurance were dominated by an interrelated group of Anglo-Saxon Protestant families from New England. In St. Paul, the German and Irish Catholic population proved more accepting of Jews. It also perhaps helped that the early Jewish settlers in St. Paul were German and entered the economic life of the city earlier in its development and with a common culture.[13]

Fannie Schanfield recalled that in Minneapolis:

> *The ads used to read, 'No Jews need apply.' It was 'no Jews allowed.' The 'For Rent' sign on the outside of the house would read, 'No Jews.' In plain, plain English: 'No Jews,' and it reminded me so much of in the South: 'No Blacks, no Jews or Dogs.' They would have it, very plain, outspoken. They didn't want us, and that's the way it was if you didn't own your house.*

Interviewees who worked within Jewish-owned businesses or lived in small towns in Minnesota often did not note antisemitism. It was those who were more actively engaged with the broader community in more urban areas who encountered it and remarked on it.

There were similarities in stories from very different locations. Anne Milavetz talked of the lack of antisemitism on the Iron Range, where she taught her neighbors how to make bagels and knishes. With a small Jewish community there, Jews knew and interacted with their non-Jewish neighbors. Rakhil Sheynkman remembered exchanging treats for holidays with her Ukrainian neighbors when she was growing up in the Ukraine before the famine.

Community

To be a community, you need gathering spaces, places to come together. Interviewees who grew up in Minnesota spoke of a variety of early gathering places, including the synagogue and the all-important kosher grocery store.

Today many of the surviving buildings that once housed synagogues have been turned into churches. Kenesseth Israel was formed in 1891 and is the oldest Orthodox congregation in Minnesota. In those early years, it served the North Minneapolis community of peddlers and small business owners, along with their families.

Many congregations and organizations grew out of Kenesseth Israel, including the predecessor to Talmud Torah of Minneapolis. As the community was largely composed of immigrants, Kenesseth Israel also offered social services such as English instruction, a medical clinic, and a shelter. Jewish homes for both children and the elderly grew out of Kenesseth Israel programs. In 1913, the congregation moved to Lyndale Avenue and created a building with two towers capped by domes, "the Lyndale Shul" remembered fondly by Shirley Sussman. The community conducted services at that location until 1948 when they sold the building to an African American church.[14]

On the other side of the river, in St. Paul, Neighborhood House became a central community presence. Zelda Katz grew up on the West Side of St. Paul and had fond memories of spending time there when she was a child.

> *Oh, I lived at the Neighborhood House. I used to go there after school . . . They had different clubs for us younger kids . . . and it was fun going after school. I still remember the head of the Neighborhood House. Constance Curry was her name, very dear lady, a very dear lady. I used to go to the Neighborhood House every day after school . . . It was a wonderful part of my life.*

Neighborhood House was started in 1897 to support immigrants in the West Side Flats with classes, a nursery school, and hot lunches. It was created in large part by established German Jews, led by members of Mount Zion Synagogue, to provide support to that first wave of new immigrants from *The Pale*. With a focus on assimilation, its offerings included classes in English, citizenship, and the practical skill of sewing. By 1903, Neighborhood House became nonsectarian; over time it continued to serve the changing immigrant population.[15]

Constance Curry directed the organization from 1918 to 1956. Prior to beginning her work there she did not know what Judaism was, nor had she met anyone Jewish. Over her nearly 40 years with Neighborhood House she developed a reputation of being sensitive to cultural values and the immigrant experience.[16]

Brochin's was an equally important institution: the first Jewish grocery store and very much a community center. The store was difficult to categorize—a grocery, a deli, and a place to purchase everything from Yiddish newspapers to prayer shawls. In Solomon Brochin's words: "On one side, I give the customer food for his stomach, on the other, I give him food for his mind."[17]

Solomon Brochin came with the immigrants of the early 1900s who were frequently fleeing either pogroms or a lengthy stint in the Russian army. In December 1906, Salman (Solomon) Brochin, age 28, and his wife, Chane (Anna), arrived in Boston on the *SS Saxonia* sailing from Liverpool. Their ultimate destination was noted as Minneapolis.[18] By 1909, Brochin is listed in the city directory as a Minneapolis confectioner with both his residence and work place located at 6th Avenue North. Work and living were closely integrated, and the whole family worked in the store.[19] The immigration manifest notes that Brochin brought $600 in a draft, and after a brief stint at salaried work, he opened his grocery store. It soon became a fixture on the North Side.

In its early days, the store was open from 6:00 a.m until 1:00 a.m. By 1924, they had moderated the hours to a mere 8:00 a.m. to midnight. A.I. Harris of the *American Jewish World* described his first visit to Brochin's back in 1909 at 11:00 at night:

> *In a far corner of the store at the rear was a group of elderly Jews with beards and* payes *gossiping and looking over Brochin's latest offerings in the line of Yiddish papers. Having absorbed all of its contents, now and then one of the men made a gesture of buying the paper, but after reconsideration, usually refolded it carefully and purchased a package of Turkish tobacco instead, or simply bade Brochin a pleasant* 'gute nacht' . . . *Mrs. Brochin was in front of the store behind a counter slicing and weighing out some corn beef for a couple of stout, 'stylish' Jewish ladies . . . Brochin himself was waiting on a group of Jewish high school students who were famished from their exertions in a nearby pool parlor, playing pool instead of conjugating Latin verbs, and they were ordering corn beef and pastroma sandwiches . . . While filling these orders, Brochin kept up a crossfire discussion with some of his cronies on some Jewish topic of the day.*[20]

In the back room, which served as the Passover store, there was a round table where Jewish leaders gathered to discuss the community problems of the day while munching on corned beef sandwiches. Local attorney Alex Kanter once brought Justice Brandeis to visit the store to demonstrate how Americanized Jews and immigrants interacted.[21]

Brochin played another important role in the immigrant community by bringing more Jews over from Russia. From 1915 to 1918 he coordinated with a Russian bank and assisted local Jews in the purchase of steamship tickets for their friends and families. Also, Brochin was known for reading and writing letters for his clientele in Russian, Polish, Ukrainian, and Yiddish.[22]

Immigration

The common thread across our interviewees was an immigration story. The first group, children of immigrants, grew up within an immigrant community. Many were very familiar with the story of how their parents came to America. Both Holocaust survivors and immigrants from the former USSR had their own immigration stories.

In 1900, more than 40% of American Jews were newcomers. Immigration declined in 1924 when immigration laws became more restrictive, and immigration quotas were put in place. The new quotas were tied to the percent each country of origin had represented of the total US population in 1890. Immigration quotas remained in effect until 1965.[23]

Fannie Schanfield and her daughter, Miriam, told of Fannie's mother and her immigration to the United States. The story unfolded, weaving back and forth between them, each correcting and adding to what the other offered. Fannie's mother had borrowed a friend's birth certificate and hence arrived with a different name from her accompanying family members. Because of her different last name, she was detained when the rest of the family was released.

"Imagine how frightened she was!" Miriam exclaimed.

Fannie nodded in agreement and proceeded:

> *If you're not picked up in four days, you're shipped back. So Shimon* [a cousin and her mother's fiancé] *promised her, 'I'll be here in four days. Don't worry.' On the fourth day, he did come, and she will tell you . . . that it was after* [the] *Fourth of July. It was on the fifth of July . . . The streets were covered with confetti, and they had a parade . . . and she asked specifically, 'Why are the streets so dirty?' Because it was the* geboyrn-tog [birthday] *of the country.*

Dorothy Brochin's parents, Solomon and Anna, left Lithuania in the wake of pogroms without telling their parents, lest they be dissuaded. Harold Wittcoff's father went AWOL from the Russian army, despite the penalty of death if he was caught. Harold's mother emigrated alone. She had joined the Communist party, so her sister sent her to America. It was not sufficient to have the fare for passage; she also had to steal across the border. A stealthy exit was a common theme from this period.

The migration experience of Holocaust survivors was quite different from that of earlier immigrants. Many came alone, their families having been murdered. Most had spent some time in DP camps and had lived in Germany, often interacting with former German soldiers as they waited to move on with their lives.

Sam Saide was almost thirteen when the war severed him from his family in Poland. At eighteen he began re-establishing his life after the war. The DP camp was full, so he was sent to a town where the burghermeister put him with a German family. He lived there for three years, learning to be a printer:

> *That was the good times already. I was playing soccer with the Germans. Every Sunday we went to another town, went home. We had beer, black beer . . . The Germans never call me* [anything] *except Samuel. Never one word no more. Not like* [it] *used to be, you know.*

During the war, the United States had been an oft-sought and seldom-obtained haven for those seeking safety. This began to change in 1945 when President Truman issued an executive order, known as the Truman Directive, that assigned immigration quotas to displaced persons. About 15,000 Jewish DPs entered the country between 1945 and 1947. The Red Scare was at its height, and the focus had shifted to Communism.

In 1948, Congress passed legislation that would admit 200,000 displaced persons, of whom 80,000 were Jewish. The others were Eastern Europeans who had been forced laborers in Germany. The bill had been carefully crafted to exclude many of the Jewish DPs who were not in the required zone as of the cutoff date, excluding the 100,000 refugees who had fled pogroms in Poland or just been released from the Soviet Union. There was also a favoring of agricultural laborers, a category which few Jews fell within.[24] Truman termed the bill "flagrantly discriminatory against Jews."[25] These policies reflected the antisemitism that was at its zenith during this period. In fact, a public opinion poll in 1948 found 53% favored admitting displaced persons to the United States, but 60% favored placing restrictions if most of them were Jews.[26] This law was finally amended in 1950 and ultimately increased admissions to 415,000. By 1952, Jewish refugees in the United States totaled more than 137,000.[27]

Antisemitism was colored by both the Rosenberg trial and the McCarthy hearings. A 1948 survey by the American Jewish Committee found 21% of Americans believed "most Jews are Communists," and more than half associated Jews with atomic spying. A 2008 study by Aviva Weingarten noted that Jews represented two-thirds of the 124 people questioned in 1952 by McCarthy's Senate Committee on Homeland Security and Government Affairs.[28]

The changing immigration laws affected Sam Saide. In September 1949, he boarded a boat in Bremerhaven, Germany and embarked for the United States.

He was twenty-two, ten years older than when the Nazis had first invaded Poland. He recalled his entry to the United States:

> *They were talking to me in English. I couldn't understand a word . . . There was some guys who understand a little bit of Polish, so I had to talk to them. They asked me if I was a Communist. Why you ask me if I was a Communist? I was in concentration camp in Germany. When was I a Communist? Communists are Russian.*

Jewish immigrants from the Soviet Union began to arrive in the 1970s, but 70% of them arrived after 1990, following the Soviet Union's collapse. When these immigrants first began to arrive, many went via a circuitous route. Upon receipt of an invitation from relatives in Israel, real or fictitious, many started their journey with Israel as the purported destination. Some chose to seek political refugee status in transit and then come to the United States.[29]

Rakhil Sheynkman's daughter, Liana Ravkin, recalled:

> *We went through couple countries. When we decided to leave at the time, they took our citizenship. And we paid for it. They told us we had to pay for it. They took from us our citizenship of Soviet Union, passports and everything. What we had is little Israeli visa because we couldn't come straight to United States. We wanted to come straight to the United States, but we had to choose between, to go to Israel or United States. At the time, we didn't plan to go to Israel, we wanted to go to the United States. We went through . . . Austria, Italy, and then to the United States . . . We have to have an interview in American embassy in Italy, and they decided if we could have refugee status, so we have to prove why.*

Later, when her mother Rakhil came over, she went directly to Minneapolis as she now had family there.

Our interviewees spanned all three Jewish immigrant groups who came over during the twentieth century. Each wave made room for the next. Each group of newcomers learned to find their place in a community that didn't always know how to incorporate them.

The existing Jewish population's desire to help the refugees fit in was colored by their fears of arousing the not-so-latent antisemitism of their neighbors. First-generation American Jews like Fannie Schanfield were instructed not to use their hands when speaking: "Fit in. Don't act Jewish."

The American Jewish community was uneasy with the horror of the Holocaust and the open question, "Could American Jews have done more?" The Holocaust and one's experience during it weren't discussed openly until decades later. Many in the Jewish community were especially uncomfortable with the sense of vulnerability it engendered in them.[30]

For immigrants from the Soviet Union, their sense of Jewish identity was shaped in response to the particular antisemitism experienced there. Having been denied the opportunity to practice Judaism earlier in life, many did not know how to do so. They didn't share the same Jewish culture that previously defined American Jewish identity.[31]

Many of our interviewees who immigrated faced difficulties common to most immigrants throughout time: learning a new language and culture, finding work that often failed to make use of their existing skills, and creating a home for the next generation—in what often proved to be more that younger generation's world than their own.

Legacy: The Next Generation

These three strands woven into today's Jewish community are, along with the whole community, still in motion, still dynamic, never static. In many ways, we have lost the elements that formed the one-time community. Some of that loss is due to the erosion of antisemitism post-World War II. As antisemitism began to decline, employment and housing opportunities allowed greater movement into the broader community. The GI Bill offered access to education, the professions, and resulting financial security. We no longer have a geographic concentration comparable to the old North Side, and few Yiddish speakers remain after the Holocaust. We live in a much more mobile world, no longer around the corner from family. Educational and career opportunities have increased migration, further fraying connections to family and community.

Looking toward the next generation, we see several trends on the horizon. With the loss of a common language and geography, Jewish communities are fostered by institutions such as synagogues, Jewish community centers, and Talmud Torah programs. Many young Jews attend Jewish camps where they may build lifelong ties with others in the community. Despite these structures for those who remain affiliated, it is entirely possible to consider oneself Jewish and live outside of a formal affiliation. Antisemitism has certainly not been eliminated; rather, it takes on new forms.

In the 2013 Pew Research survey on Jewish attitudes, 93% of those born between 1914 and 1927 considered themselves Jewish by religion. This dropped to 68% among Millennials, born after 1980. Twenty-two percent of Jews described themselves as having no religion.[32] So, what comes next?

Intermarriage is one theme that came up over the course of our interviews. One interviewee, a mother whose daughter had married a non-Jew, maintained contact with her daughter, but her husband withdrew for several years. He would neither see their daughter nor welcome her to their home. The mother recounted how one day he burst into tears and called out for their daughter. When she invited their daughter and son-in-law over, father and daughter happily renewed their relationship. When their second daughter married a non-Jew, they made a small wedding, having come to terms with this challenge in how they viewed their family.

Another interviewee referred to her young grandchildren, rather fondly, as "the little *shikselas*." Sometimes interviewees spoke of choosing their words carefully, not wanting to alienate their children's or grandchildren's spouses, and working hard to accept a reality they had not anticipated. And they wondered about their legacy. What would be retained? What would be valued? Would these grandchildren who grew up in a very different tradition value their Jewish heritage?

Of those Jews marrying since 2000, almost 60% have a non-Jewish spouse, an increase from 17% before 1970. As restrictions have fallen, intermarriage and assimilation have begun to break down barriers and reshape identity. Jewish identity is being redefined for grandchildren who may have only one Jewish parent and may grow up with multiple traditions. How much of the heritage will be preserved remains an open question.

Another very different theme that came up through the elders was about children and grandchildren reclaiming and renewing ties with Judaism. This was especially true of immigrants from the former Soviet Union who took great pleasure in this reconnection with a heritage they had been denied. Rakhil *kvelled* over her grandsons, who are receiving a Jewish education, especially her oldest grandson who led them through the Passover Seder.

The children and grandchildren I interviewed expressed deep respect for their elders and pride in their history. Their family relationships were strong, and they built their own lives upon the stories of their parents and grandparents. Walter Schwarz's children shared a sense of social activism they attributed to their parents' experience in the Holocaust. His daughter spoke of the trauma of the Holocaust as a family trauma. Hanna Lyon's daughter, a teacher, talked of how her mother's Holocaust experience affected the way she taught Holocaust awareness to her students. Both of Hanna's daughters spoke of sensing the pain their mother had submerged. The Wittcoffs' son, Ralph, attributed his career as a community organizer to his parents' involvement in Labor Zionism. He recognized his exposure to their ideals and love of learning as formative elements in his life. Ralph's daughter also absorbed a deep curiosity about the world and her grandparents' passion for travel. Liana Ravkin was proud of her mother Rakhil Sheynkman's accomplishments during the war and valued the history Rakhil had shared with her through food, song, and, of course, story.

Fannie Schanfield gave her daughter, Miriam, a lifetime membership in Hadassah on her eighteenth birthday. The two were very close, and Miriam looked to her mother's community engagement with admiration. Fannie's legacy of an active community life is also continued by a granddaughter who studied to be a rabbi, a source of great pride to Fannie.

Many of those I interviewed took great pride in Israel, and I wondered whether this carried over to more youthful populations within the Jewish community, particularly as Israeli policies have come under fire on college campuses. Interestingly, in 2013, the Pew Research Center reported no evidence of declining attachment, with 70% reporting an attachment to Israel. A more recent study of Birthright applicants, one-third of whom come from intermarried families, took a look at the younger segment split into those who went on the trip and those who didn't, over the period of the Israel-Hamas war. In fact, the sense of connection to Israel increased for both groups. While support was substantial across all groups, those who defined themselves as liberal showed a somewhat lower level of support, but a greater proportional increase.[33]

So what defines our Jewish community across generations? Fannie proposed Yiddishkeit as the unifying concept. The way Fannie defined it may have changed somewhat, but it still is a term big enough to embrace the way many of us define being Jewish. Responses to The Pew Study identified those qualities as: remembering the Holocaust, leading an ethical life, working for justice and equality, being intellectually curious, caring about Israel, and having a good sense of humor. Lower on the list were the more traditional criteria of being part of a Jewish community, observing Jewish law, and eating Jewish foods. Critical assessment is welcomed, with 89% feeling it was acceptable to be critical of Israel. Being Jewish is more often defined culturally than religiously, with more than two-thirds (68%) believing one can be Jewish and not believe in God. It's a big tent we pitch. While Fannie's Yiddishkeit was of a more affiliated variety, I see many of the same threads she espoused in the survey findings. Her prayer shawl of tzedakah and mitzvah still wraps the Jewish community in its values.

Final Thoughts

This was a project that grew in scope far beyond what I originally anticipated. The simple act of asking about a person's life story creates a powerful connection and, for me, a deeper appreciation of a community's complexity. Most of my interviewees were in their 90s when I spoke with them, and many are no longer alive. As I began to pull together their stories, I often wished that I could go back to follow up on a thread that was seemingly insignificant at the time, but grew in importance to me. I've attended many of their shivas and funerals and been genuinely saddened at their loss. These people touched me in surprising ways.

As for identity and legacy, there were no simple answers. Some interviewees were defined by relationships, others by their early exposure to Jewish heritage, some by antisemitism, and still others by their community's embrace. Story was important to interviewees as a vehicle for sharing their experiences.

Each group had similarities within. Those who grew up in early immigrant communities had fond memories of these communities. Their identity was defined by the culture in which they were nurtured.

Holocaust survivors found their way to the US and began to rebuild their lives. Most were in their twenties and thirties, having survived as forced labor for the Nazis. They began to form new families as they learned English and entered mainstream American society. Those early years were no doubt challenging. Discussion of their experience was not encouraged by American Jews who were ill at ease with the subject of the Holocaust.

Elder interviewees who came from the Soviet Union arrived later in life, following their children. They were less likely to learn English at this stage in life. They took pride in their children, who were rediscovering Judaism and quickly acclimating to American society. Though their migration was less about themselves and more about their children, their presence offered an important link to the history from which their families grew.

I was especially struck by how my story as an American secular Jew fit within this larger community. Each thread bore a connection to my own family history. I found myself embracing each history, feeling it was my own as well.

It was an honor to play a role in sharing these stories with the larger community, and I am deeply grateful to each of my interviewees for sharing their stories with me.

Acknowledgments

There are many people who played a significant role in assuring the completion of this project and ultimately this book.

When I first spoke to Carol Kvasnik at Sholom and in an impulsive moment suggested the idea of interviewing residents, I had no expectation of it coming to fruition. My impulse was translated to reality by Carol's recognition of possibility. My subsequent meeting with Rabbi Shalom Reznik-Bell and the Sholom staff and program directors gave it legs. A special thank you to Jen Zinnel, Pam Ulseth-Gusdal, and Helen Gurevich who recommended interview subjects and assisted in coordinating those interviews. In addition, I am especially grateful for Helen's assistance with translation between Russian and English.

This book, the artwork, and the interviews would not exist without the key contributors, my interviewees, both elders and their participating family members. Each interviewee contributed their story and shared their experience openly. There is a connection forged during an interview. For the interviewees, it was shaped by an expression of interest and a value placed on their story; for me it was shaped by the opportunity to step into someone else's experience and to share it with others. Interviewees and family who made this book possible include Bernice Gordon; Zelda Katz; Boris Lerner; Yevgeniy Mazo; Anne Milavetz; Trudy Rappaport; Sam Saide; Shirley Sussman; Hanna Lyon and her family members Susan Lyon, Deborah Lyon, Rachel Lutchen, and Shawnee Elliott; Dorothy and Harold Wittcoff and their family members Ralph Wittcoff and Wendy Downes; Fannie Scharfield and her daughter Miriam Kieffer; Walter Schwarz and his family members Sylvia, Dan, and Karen Schwarz; and Rakhil Sheynkman and her daughter Liana Ravkin.

Katherine Tane, the former director of the Jewish Historical Society of the Upper Midwest (JHSUM), provided guidance as I wrote grants and developed a protocol for interviews. She also offered additional ideas, opening the path that led me to the next generation.

Carla Vogel played an important role in our interviewing and brought a different sensibility into the room. Our very different personalities, mine driven, hers much more fluid, proved beneficial in the process of interviewing. When I would get stuck on where to go next, Carla was likely to invite our interviewee to share their favorite Yiddish song. As they sang for us, a sense of comfort filled the room, easing the interview forward.

The interviews were financed in part with funds provided to Sholom by the State of Minnesota through the Minnesota Historical Society from the Arts & Cultural Heritage Fund. When this book was ready for publication, the Minnesota

Historical Society once again offered their support through the State of Minnesota legacy funds, providing funding to the Jewish Historical Society of the Upper Midwest to make this book a reality. Their support allowed us to capture these often poignant and powerful stories.

The JHSUM was an important partner throughout this project, from their guidance as I completed the interviews to their support in publishing the book itself. JHSUM Executive Director Robin Doroshow, together with the Board, played an important role in ushering the project to its next stage, sharing my belief in the value of telling the important stories of our community.

The community at large was in many ways the impetus for this book. After I completed the interviews and artwork, I began showing the work and speaking to organizations within the Twin Cities. As I played video and shared story, I realized from responses that another piece was needed, a written document. I had begun part of that documentation as I did the interviews and created the artwork, writing about the process within my blog Layers of the Onion. From my interactions with the community I realized that it was time to explore the narrative possibilities more deeply and began developing this book.

As the book took shape, several people offered fresh perspectives as they reviewed drafts and offered suggestions. My dear friend Dora Zaidenweber's understanding of the broader Jewish community informed my efforts and identified gaps to fill. Lucy Rose Fischer provided me with her invaluable perspective as a fellow artist and writer. Meryll Page brought her experience as a writer and her deep knowledge of Jewish history and the Soviet Jewish experience. Annette Atkins applied her lens as a historian with a focus on social and cultural history.

Margie Newman graciously lent her assistance in helping me to capture the Yiddish phrases that rolled off the tongue of many of my interviewees. Nicole Messinger Post provided the ever-valuable perspective of an editor and Rachel Holscher patiently helped me through the many decisions of design, layout, and publication.

My husband, Martin Arend, followed this effort from beginning to end. He heard about the interviews when I returned home from each one, spilling over with excitement. He listened to the endless repetition as I transcribed and edited video, and he was my first reader, long before the book was polished enough for the eyes of others.

My sister, Andrea Weinberg-Chestnut, played an essential role in editing, providing feedback and the occasional prod to keep going. There were many places along the way where I could have easily faltered. Having the support of my sister was invaluable. We often talked of how much our late mother would have loved the idea of us working together on this effort. I had read sections of this to our mother, and she had talked of how much she would love to read it in print. While that never came to pass in her lifetime, her presence was deeply felt throughout.

Author Biography

Susan Weinberg is an artist, writer, and genealogist with a deep love of story. Through artwork, oral history, and text, Susan shares stories of Jewish heritage. She believes it is through story that we understand our common connections. This book grew out of that deeply-felt belief.

When Susan left a career in finance, she began to volunteer with the Jewish Historical Society of the Upper Midwest, providing talks on Jewish genealogy. She soon moved that interest into an artistic realm with a show of artwork about her personal family history. Ultimately that work connected her with Sholom where the oral history project that underlies this book began.

Susan's interest in heritage took her overseas to study Yiddish at the Vilnius Yiddish Institute and to visit her ancestral towns in Belarus, the Ukraine, and Poland. It fed artwork on the Holocaust history of Lithuania and took her on an artistic journey into the former Jewish community of Radom, Poland. She then returned closer to home where she began the Jewish Identity and Legacy Project, a series of oral histories, which ultimately unfolded into the artwork and story that comprise this book.

Susan lives in Minnesota with her husband, Martin Arend. She paints, writes, and speaks about her many interests, sharing stories with the community about the rich history that underlies it. Susan works out of her studio in NE Minneapolis where you can see some of the paintings found in this book.

Glossary

alef-beys. (Yiddish) Jewish alphabet. Also *aleph bes* and, in Hebrew, *alef bet* or *aleph bet.*

aliyah. (Hebrew, Yiddish) An honorary role during the synagogue service, such as being called to recite the blessings over the Torah.

Babi Yar. A ravine in the Kiev region and a site of massacres carried out by German forces and local collaborators during WWII.

balalaika. A Russian stringed instrument with a triangular body and three strings.

benching licht. Lighting and blessing candles on special occasions such as Shabbat.

beshert. (Yiddish) Fated. Intended. Meant to be.

Birobidzhan. An administrative division of southeast Russia, in eastern Siberia, that was colonized by Jews in 1928 and largely agricultural.

Birthright. A nonprofit educational organization that sponsors free ten-day heritage trips to Israel for young people of ages eighteen to twenty-six.

bubbe. (Yiddish) Grandmother.

burghermeister. Chairman of the executive council in German towns; literally means "master of the citizens."

Chaim Weitzman. A Zionist leader and Israeli statesman who became the first President of Israel.

challah. A special bread used on Shabbat and Jewish holidays.

chazan. (Yiddish) Ordained Jewish clergy person whose role includes singing liturgical music and leading prayers at a synagogue; also called *cantor.*

cheder. A school for Jewish children that teaches Hebrew and religious knowledge.

concentration camp. A camp established by the Nazis during WWII to hold those they considered "undesirables" such as Jews, gypsies, homosexuals, etc. The conditions were such that many died of starvation and typhoid. Some camps were also extermination camps with gas chambers. Auschwitz ("Oswiecm" in Polish) and Majdanek were both extermination camps.

Diego Velasquez. A Spanish painter in the court of King Philip IV. One of the most important painters of the 17th century.

displaced persons (DP) camp. Temporary facility for persons who were displaced from their homes. After WWII, DP camps were established in Germany, Italy, and Austria for survivors of the Nazi concentration camps and for others who had been displaced by the war.

Es shoyn, es. (Yiddish) Literally means "Eat already, eat."

fleishig. (Yiddish) Meat, thus not mixed with dairy under kosher dietary rules.

flick. (Yiddish) pluck.

geboyrn-tog. (Yiddish) birthday.

gefilte fish. A dish made from a poached mixture of deboned, seasoned, and ground fish, usually carp, whitefish, or pike.

Hadassah. A Jewish women's organization.

Holocaust. The mass slaughter of six million Jews as well as other targeted groups by the Nazis during WWII, referred to by many within the Jewish community as the Shoah.

Holodomor. Man-made famine imposed by Stalin from 1932 to 1933 that killed 2.5–7.5 million Ukrainians.

Israel-Hamas war. The fifty-day military conflict in 2014 between Israel and Hamas involving the Gaza strip.

Juan Bautista Martinez del Mazo. A 17th-century Spanish Baroque painter of portraits and landscapes who was a follower and son-in-law of Velasquez.

Juden raus. (German) Jews out.

kikhl. (Yiddish) cookie.

Kindertransport. A World War II rescue effort focused on bringing children from Germany and German-occupied territories to safety.

kippah. (Hebrew) brimless cloth cap worn by observant Jews; also *yarmulke.*

knish. A savory hand pie, either baked or fried, that contains any of a variety of fillings such as meat, potatoes, spinach, cheese, or other vegetables.

Kristallnacht. November 9–10, 1938 was the Night of Broken Glass, an anti-Jewish pogrom throughout Nazi Germany, Austria, and German-occupied territories; carried out by stormtroopers and German civilians, it was supported by German authorities.

kugel. A baked pudding or casserole made with egg noodles or potato.

kvelled. (Yiddish) took pride in.

Labor Zionism. The left wing of the Zionist movement, it supported the creation of kibbutzim and believed a Jewish state could only be created through the efforts of the Jewish working class settling in Palestine to create a Progressive Jewish society.

leckach. Traditional Eastern European Jewish honey cake.

Leningrad front. The Soviet unit charged with defending Leningrad (now St. Petersburg). They stopped the German army at the outskirts of Leningrad, though the siege continued for two-and-a-half years.

Louis Brandeis. The first Jew to be named to the US Supreme Court, he served from 1916–1939 and was known as a strong defender of freedom of speech and privacy rights.

Lozn sha. (Yiddish) Be quiet.

Majdanek. A concentration and extermination camp outside of the city of Lublin, Poland, largely intact because the Germans left quickly as the Soviets approached.

McCarthy hearings. The series of hearings run by Senator Joe McCarthy in the 1950s to identify communist sympathizers in the US.

milchig. (Yiddish) dairy, thus not to be mixed with meat under kosher dietary rules.

mitzvah. (Hebrew, Yiddish) literally means "commandment;" commonly used to mean "good deed."

Oswiecim. Polish name for Auschwitz, a concentration and extermination camp near Krakow, Poland.

The Pale. Area in Eastern Europe where Jews were required to live.

Passover Seder. A Jewish ritual feast to mark the holiday of Passover which celebrates the release of the Israelites from slavery in Egypt and their journey to freedom.

payes. (Hebew) sidelocks worn for religious purposes by traditional Jewish males. Also *payos.*

pogrom. An organized massacre, typically against Jews in Russia or Eastern Europe.

Red Scare. promotion by a state or society of a fear of Communist infiltration, the first Red Scare in the US followed WWI; the second was in the 1950s.

Ritchie Boy. US special military intelligence officers with German language skills who interrogated German prisoners.

Rosenberg trial. The 1951 trial of Communist Party members Ethel and Julius Rosenberg, for selling nuclear secrets to Russia, ended in conviction and execution.

Shabbat/Shabbos. The Jewish Sabbath. *Shabbat* is Hebrew and *Shabbos* is Yiddish.

shiksa. (Yiddish) non-Jewish girl.

shiksela. (Yiddish) non-Jewish little girls, diminutive form *shiksa.*

shoykhet. (Yiddish) kosher butcher.

shraybn. (Yiddish) write.

Shrayb es arop. (Yiddish) write it down.

shtiebel. (Yiddish) a place for communal Jewish prayer, literally means "little room" or "little house."

shtetl. (Yiddish) a small Jewish town in Eastern Europe.

shul. (Yiddish) Synagogue. Also *schul.*

Stalingrad battle. A major battle in which Nazi Germany battled the Soviets for control of Stalingrad, ultimately ending in the surrender of Axis forces after five months of warfare.

tallesim. (Yiddish) Prayer shawls.

tallitot. (Hebrew) Prayer shawls.

Talmud Torah. A school that teaches about Judaism.

tikkun olam. (Hebrew, Yiddish) Human action to repair the world, a focal concept in Judaism.

Truman Directive. An executive order by President Truman in 1945 to allocate the existing immigration quotas to displaced persons. This was followed by more substantial laws passed by Congress that opened up greater immigration access to survivors.

tzedakah. (Hebrew, Yiddish) Literally means "justice;" commonly used to mean "charity."

yarmulke. (Yiddish) See *Kippah*, above.

Yiddishkeit. (Yiddish) The Jewish way of life, customs, and practice.

yontif. (Yiddish) Special day. Holiday.

Paintings by Susan Weinberg

Sleeping with the Chickens, from the story of Shirley Sussman 2
Lozn Sha, from the story of Shirley Sussman 5
Alef-Beys, from the story of Bernice Gordon 8
Yiddishkeit, from the story of Fannie Schanfield 10
Fire, Light, and Legacy, from the story of Fannie Schanfield 15
Grandma Zelda, from the story of Zelda Katz 16
Making Knishes, from the story of Anne Milavetz 21
Body and Soul, from the story of Dorothy Brochin Wittcoff 22
A Matter of Chemistry, from the story of Harold Wittcoff 29
Everything Stopped, from the story of Hanna Lyon 32
Postcard from New Ulm, from the story of Trudy Rappaport 36
Bricks for Bread, from the story of Sam Saide 45
Bessie Sends Greetings, from the story of Walter Schwarz 46
From Her Mother, from the story of Rakhil Sheynkman 59
Fallen Leaves, from the story of Boris Lerner 60
Unchained Legacy, from the story of Yevgeniy Mazo 67

Artwork Notes

All paintings are either 24"x 30" if landscape or 30" x 24" if portrait
Acrylic on canvas, except *Bessie Sends Greetings*—mixed media
Completion dates range from 2011-2017
More information on these paintings and other artwork can be found at studio409art.com

Bibliography

Interviews

All interviews, both transcripts and recordings, are housed at the Nathan and Theresa Berman Upper Midwest Jewish Archives, University of Minnesota, Minneapolis, MN and were done at Sholom facilities in Minneapolis and St. Paul, Minnesota.

Anne Milavetz. By Susan Weinberg and Carla Vogel. March 22, 2011.

Bernice Gordon. By Susan Weinberg and Carla Vogel. August 10, 2010 and September 3, 2010.

Boris Lerner. By Susan Weinberg. Translated by Helen Gurevich. February 23, 2011.

Dorothy Brochin Wittcoff, Harold Wittcoff, Ralph Wittcoff, Wendy Downes. By Susan Weinberg and Carla Vogel. June 6, 2012.

Fannie Schanfield. By Susan Weinberg and Carla Vogel. January 29,2011 and February 6, 2011.

Fannie Schanfield and Miriam Kieffer. By Susan Weinberg and Carla Vogel. January 29, 2012.

Gertrude Rappaport. By Susan Weinberg. March 30, 2011.

Hanna Lyon, Deborah Lyon, Shawnee Elliott, Susan Lyon, Rachel Lutchen, By Susan Weinberg and Carla Vogel. April 22, 2012.

Rakhil Sheynkman. By Susan Weinberg. Translated by Helen Gurevich. March 30, 2011.

Rakhil Sheynkman and Liana Ravkin (also Translator). By Susan Weinberg and Carla Vogel. August 9, 2012.

Sam Saide. By Susan Weinberg and Carla Vogel. March 29, 2011.

Shirley Sussman. By Susan Weinberg and Carla Vogel. January 19, 2011.

Walter Schwarz. By Susan Weinberg and Carla Vogel. April 26, 2011.

Walter Schwarz, Dan and Karen Schwarz, Sylvia Schwarz. By Susan Weinberg and Carla Vogel March 31, 2011.

Yevgeniy Mazo. By Susan Weinberg. Translated by Helen Gurevich. February 23, 2011.

Zelda Katz. By Susan Weinberg and Carla Vogel. February 22, 2011.

Other Sources

Belluck, Pam. "For Better Social Skills Scientists Recommend a Little Chekhov," Well Blog. *New York Times*. October 3, 2013. Accessed December 10, 2015. http://well.blogs.nytimes.com/2013/10/03/i-know-how-youre-feeling-i-read-chekhov/

Brochin, Salman and Chane. *SS Saxonia* Passenger Manifest. December 8, 1906. Stamped page 69, line 11–12. *Passenger Lists of Vessels Arriving at Boston, Massachusetts, 1891–1943*. Records of the Immigration and Naturalization Service 1787–2004. Record Group 8. National Archives Microfilm Publication T843, roll 102. NAI Number 4319742.

Brochin, Solomon. *Minneapolis City Directory Collection 1859–1922*. 1909.299. Hennepin County Library James K. Hosmer Special Collection. Accessed April 3, 2017. http://box2.nmtvault.com/Hennepin2/

Bush, Lawrence. "McCarthyism and the Jews." *Jewish Currents*. May 1, 2011. Accessed March 6, 2016. http://jewishcurrents.org/may-2-mccarthyism-and-the-jews-5111

Davis, Mark. "How World War II Shaped Modern Russia." *Euronews*. April 5, 2015. Accessed December 24, 2016. http://www.euronews.com/2015/05/04/how-world-war-ii-shaped-modern-russia

Dinnerstein, Leonard. *America and the Survivors of the Holocaust*. New York: Columbia University Press, 1982.

Feinstein, Stephen C. "Soviet Jewish Immigrants in Minneapolis and St. Paul Attitudes and Reactions to Life in America." In *Studies of the Third Wave: Recent Migration of Soviet Jews to the United States*, edited by Dan Jacobs and Ellen Frankel Paul, 57–75. Boulder, CO: Westview Press. 1981.

Fivish, Robyn, Jennifer G. Bohanek, and Marshall Duke. "The Intergenerational Self: Subjective Perspective and Family History." *Self Continuity: Individual and Collective Perspectives*, edited by Fabio Sani.Mahwah, NJ: Erlbaum, 2008. Accessed Dec 10, 2015. http://www.psychology.emory.edu/cognition/fivush/lab/FivushLabWebsite/papers/intergenself.pdf

Goldblum, Kenneth. "A Russian Connection: A Philatelic Adventure." Joseph Brochin Collection. Box 18. Nathan and Theresa Berman Upper Midwest Jewish Archives.

Harris, A.I. "Local Jewish Personalities." *American Jewish World*. September 4, 1924.

Hobbie, Ann S. "Much Good Work Must Here Be Done: The Neighborhood House and Eastern European Jews." Macalester College, St. Paul, MN. April 19, 1988. Independent Researcher Papers. Nathan and Theresa Berman Upper Midwest Jewish Archives, University of Minnesota.

Kanter, Alex. "I Knew Brandeis." *The Jewish Veteran*. date unknown. 6. Ben Brochin Collection. Nathan and Theresa Berman Upper Midwest Jewish Archives, University of Minnesota.

Kliger, Sam. "Russian-Jewish Immigrants in the U.S: Social Portrait, Challenges, and AJC Involvement." Accessed December 10, 2015. http://www.ajcrussian.org/site/apps/nlnet/content2.aspx?c=chLMK3PKLsF&b=7718799&ct=11713359

Lewin, Rhoda. *Jewish Community of North Minneapolis*. South Carolina: Arcadia Publishing, 2001.

Migration Policy Institute. "Major U.S. Immigration Laws: 1790-Present." Washington, D.C.: Migration Policy Institute. March 2013. Accessed December 22, 2016. http://www.migrationpolicy.org/research/timeline-1790

McWilliams, Carey. "The Curious Twin." *Common Ground*. Autumn 1946. 61–66.

Pew Research Center's Religion & Public Life Project. "A Portrait of Jewish Americans." Washington, D.C: Pew Research Center, October 1, 2013. Accessed April 24, 2016. http://www.pewforum.org/2013/10/01/jewish-american-beliefs-attitudes-culture-survey

Rahjavendran, Beena. "'A force to be reckoned with' wherever people needed her." Minneapolis Star Tribune. August 11, 2016. Accessed August 12, 2016. http://www.startribune.com/obituary-dorothy-wittcoff-social-worker-teacher-and-world-traveler/389806671

Sasson, Theodore Saxe, Leonard, Shain, Michelle. "How Do Young American Jews Feel About Israel?" Tablet. February 24, 2015. Accessed April 24, 2016. http://www.tabletmag.com/scroll/189210/how-do-young-american-jews-feel-about-israel

Sherman, Amy. "From Refugees to New Americans: How Holocaust Survivors Became Jewish Americans in the Twin Cities." May 18, 1994. Independent Researchers Papers. Nathan and Theresa Berman Upper Midwest Jewish Archives, University of Minnesota.

Storhoff, Marg. "Hadassah Called 'Way of Life.'" *Minneapolis Tribune*. May 21, 1967.

United States Holocaust Memorial Museum. "United States Policy Toward Jewish Refugees, 1941–1952." *Holocaust Encyclopedia*. Washington D.C.: United States Holocaust Memorial Museum. Accessed December 10, 2015. http://www.ushmm.org/wlc/en/article.php?ModuleId=10007094

Weber, Laura E. "Gentiles Preferred, Minneapolis Jews and Employment 1920–1950." *Minnesota History*, Spring 1991. 167–182.

Weber, Laura. "Kenesseth Israel Congregation, St. Louis Park." *Mnopedia*. Published January 23, 2014, updated September 2, 2015. Accessed March 6, 2016. http://www.mnopedia.org/group/kenesseth-israel-congregation-st-louis-park

Notes

1. Robyn Fivish, Jennifer G. Bohanek, and Marshall Duke, "The Intergenerational Self," 131–144.
2. Belluck, "For Better Social Skills Scientists Recommend a Little Chekhov."

One Foot in Both Worlds

3. Rhoda Lewin, *Jewish Community of North Minneapolis*, 195.
4. Storhoff, Marg, "Hadassah Called Way of Life."
5. Minneapolis City Directory of 1909, 299.
6. Beena Rahjavendran, ""A Force to be Reckoned With . . ."
7. Cary McWilliams, "Minneapolis: The Curious Twin," 61.

Jews from the USSR

8. Mark Davis, "How World War II Shaped Modern Russia."

The Living Archive

9. Storhoff, "Haddassah Called . . . "
10. Laura Weber, "Gentiles Preferred," 174.
11. Ibid., 180.
12. McWilliams, "Minneapolis: The Curious Twin," 61.
13. Ibid., 62–63.
14. Laura Weber, "Kenesseth Israel Congregation . . ."
15. "Ann S. Hobbie, "Much Good . . . ," 19–20.
16. Ibid., 55–77.
17. Kenneth Goldblum, "A Russian Connection . . . ," 1.
18. Salman and Chane Brochin, *SS Saxonia,* Passenger Manifest of December 8, 1906.
19. Minneapolis City Directory of 1909, 299.
20. A.I. Harris, "Local Jewish Personalities-Solomon Brochin."
21. Alex Kanter, "I Knew Brandeis."
22. Kenneth Goldblum, "A Russian Connection: A Philatelic Adventure," 3.
23. Migration Policy Institute, "Major U.S. Immigration Laws: 1790–Present."
24. Dinnerstein, Leonard, *America and the survivors of the Holocaust*, 166–172.
25. United States Holocaust Memorial Museum, "United States Policy . . ."
26. Leonard Dinnerstein, *America and the Survivors of the Holocaust*, 176.
27. United States Holocaust Memorial Museum, "United States Policy . . ."
28. Lawrence Bush, "McCarthyism and the Jews."
29. Sam Kliger, "Russian-Jewish Immigrants in the U.S."
30. Amy Sherman, "From Refugees to New Americans."
31. Stephen C. Feinstein, "Soviet Jewish Immigrants in Minneapolis and St. Paul," 72–74.

Legacy: The Next Generation

32. Pew Research Center's Religion & Public Life Project Center, "A Portrait of Jewish Americans."
33. Theodore Sasson, Leonard Saxe, Michelle Shain, "How Do Young American Jews Feel About Israel?"

Index

Antisemitism, xiii, 1, 20, 27, 30, 51, 53, 55, 57-58, 63, 66, 68-70, 74-77, 81
Auschwitz, also Oswiecim, 33, 43, 50, 55
Benching licht, 14
Berman Upper Midwest Jewish Archives, 12, 69
Beth Jacob, 17, 18
Birthright, 79
B'nai Abraham, 19
B'nai Emet, 13, 14
Bohanek, Jennifer, ix
Brandeis, Louis, Supreme Court justice, 23, 72
Brochin, Anna or Chane, 23, 72
Brochin, Solomon or Salman, 23, 25, 72-73
Brochin's, store, 69, 72
Camp Ritchie, 48
Displaced Person, also DP, 74
Displaced Persons Camps, 24, 31, 39, 74
Duke, Marshall, ix
Emory's Center for Myth and Ritual in American Life, ix
Federation of Women Teachers of Minneapolis, 70
First-Generation Americans, 10, 75
Fivish, Robyn, ix
Gordon, Bernice, 8-9
Hadassah, 11, 20, 30, 69, 78
Harris, A.I., 72
Holocaust, x, xiii, 31, 33, 37, 50-51, 61, 69, 73-74, 76-79, 81
Holocaust survivors, also survivors, x, xiii, 31, 33, 40, 50, 61, 68, 73-74, 81
Holodomor, 53
Humphrey, Hubert, 70
Immigration, 1, 28, 31, 38, 55, 68-69, 72-75
Intergenerational Self, ix
Iron Range, also Range, 19-20, 70
Jewish Historical Society of the Upper Midwest, x, 101
Kanter, Alex, 72
Katz, Zelda, 16-18, 71
Kenesseth Israel, 71
Kiev, 53-56, 58
Kindertransport, 33
Kristallnacht, 38
Labor Zionism, 28, 78
Leningrad, 63, 66
Lerner, Boris, 60-63
Line 5, xii, 58
Lyndale Shul, 4, 71
Lyon, Hanna, 32-35, 37, 78
Majdanek, 55
Mazo, Yevgeniy, 65-67
McCarthy hearings, 74
McWilliams, Carey, 27, 70
Milavetz, Anne, 19-21, 70
Minsk, 65, 66
Mogilev Podolsk, 61, 62
Neighborhood House, 71
New Home Club, 40
North Side, 1, 23, 40, 72, 77
Pew Research, also Pew Study, 77, 79
Podol, 53
Pogrom, xii, 23, 69, 72-74
Rappaport, Trudy, 36-41
Red Cross letters, 33-35
Red Scare, 74
Ritchie Boy(s), 48-49
Rosenberg trial, 74
Saide, Sam, 43-45, 74-75
Schanfield, Fannie, 10-15, 69, 70, 73, 75, 78
Schwartz, Simon, 13
Schwarz, Walter, 46-49, 78
Shanghai, 38-39, 41
Sheynkman, Rakhil, 53-59, 70, 75, 78
Sholom, ix-xi, 9, 19, 33, 35, 37, 43, 68-69, 101
Silvers, Osias, 13
Soviet Union, x, xi, xiii, 51, 54-55, 57-58, 68, 74-76, 78, 81
Speaking Jewish, also spoke Jewish, xii-xiii, 6-7
Stalingrad, 54
Sumner School, 6
Sussman, Shirley, 2-7, 71
Theresienstadt, 49
Truman Directive, 74
USSR, xiii, 51, 62, 69, 73
Weingarten, Aviva, 74
Weitzman, Chaim, 23
Wittcoff, Dorothy Brochin, 22-25, 73
Wittcoff, Harold, 27-29, 73
Yiddish, xiii, 1, 6, 9, 11, 23, 25, 56, 58, 61, 68, 72-73, 77
Yiddishkeit, xiii, 10-12, 30, 79

About my Partners

The Jewish Historical Society of the Upper Midwest shared their expertise and guidance in oral histories and assisted in the publication of this book. Established in 1984, the JHSUM works to promote the vitality and continuity of Jewish culture in the Upper Midwest, preserving, interpreting and sharing the stories of communities of the past with communities of the present.

As a 501(c)3 membership organization JHSUM serves a community of scholars, educators, students, genealogists, family historians, and the general public. Its archives are housed at the University of Minnesota's Nathan and Theresa Berman Upper Midwest Jewish Archives. You can learn more about JHSUM and its exhibitions and publications at jhsum.org and about the archives at lib.umn.edu/umja.

Sholom originally recognized the potential in this project and facilitated the interviews with elders within its community of residents. Sholom works in partnership with the community to support adults in need across the continuum of care, to live life fully in a Jewish environment where all are welcome. With more than 100 years of service, Sholom offers campus-based programs in Minneapolis/St. Louis Park and St. Paul as well as community-based services across the metro area.

Sholom recognizes the elderly are individuals with psychological, emotional, spiritual, social, and physical needs and works with individuals and their families to find the most comfortable and enjoyable living arrangements. You can learn more about Sholom at sholom.com.